Viral BS

Viral BS

Medical Myths and
Why We Fall for Them

DR. SEEMA YASMIN

Johns Hopkins University Press

Baltimore

Johns Hopkins University Press
2715 North Charles Street
Baltimore, Maryland 21218-4363
www.press.jhu.edu

Library of Congress Cataloging-in-Publication Data

Names: Yasmin, Seema, 1982– author.
Title: Viral BS : medical myths and why we fall for them / Dr. Seema Yasmin.
Description: Baltimore : Johns Hopkins University Press, 2021. | Includes index.
Identifiers: LCCN 2020018587 | ISBN 9781421440408 (hardcover) | ISBN 9781421440415 (ebook)
Subjects: LCSH: Medical misconceptions—Miscellanea.
Classification: LCC R729.9 .Y37 2020 | DDC 610—dc23
LC record available at https://lccn.loc.gov/2020018587

A catalog record for this book is available from the British Library.

*Special discounts are available for bulk purchases of this book. For more information,
please contact Special Sales at specialsales@press.jhu.edu.*

Johns Hopkins University Press uses environmentally friendly book materials, including recycled
text paper that is composed of at least 30 percent post-consumer waste, whenever possible.

CONTENTS

INTRODUCTION

One morning in the fall of 2014, a woman walked into a pediatrician's office in Texas. Six thousand miles away, across the Atlantic Ocean, an Ebola outbreak was spreading through Sierra Leone, Guinea, and Liberia. The virus had infected thousands of West Africans and killed nearly 5,000 people.

In Texas, the woman asked the pediatrician to give her daughter a vaccine to protect against Ebola.

"There is no vaccine for Ebola," the doctor replied. "And even if we had one, your daughter wouldn't need it. She's not at risk of getting Ebola."

The mother wasn't convinced. She asked again. Ebola was killing people and her daughter needed the Ebola vaccine. This time the pediatrician shifted the conversation away from Ebola to a far deadlier disease: flu. Flu kills upward of 40,000 Americans every year, most of them children. Some years the death count doubles and creeps past the 80,000 mark.

"I can't give your daughter a vaccine for Ebola," the pediatrician said, "because an Ebola vaccine doesn't exist. But it is flu season and I can give your daughter the flu vaccine."

"Flu vaccine?!" the mother scoffed. "I don't believe in those things!" She stormed out of the doctor's office.

We are strange, complicated, irrational animals. Our brains process information at a rate of a billion billion calculations per second, a number so large it's known as an exaFLOP, a processing capability unmatched by any supercomputer.

Our ability to process such an extraordinary amount of information so quickly doesn't mean we do it sensibly. We are more likely to die in a car crash but more scared of flying on a plane; more likely to die from flu but more scared of Ebola.

Sometimes the inputs don't make sense. In a murky world full of uncertainty, we fill in the knowledge gaps, color in our fears with theories and stories

1

that help us make sense of the unknowns. Facts are boring. Flu deaths and car crashes are mundane. Ebola, a plane falling out of the sky, those stories are sensational.

The stories we tell ourselves, even the ones that scare the pants off of us—that our baby girl in central Texas could seep blood from every orifice because of a viral hemorrhagic fever, that vaccines mandated by schools could shrink our children's brains—are sticky stories that we remember.

Stories brimming with highs and lows, tension, exquisite detail, and suspense stimulate the release of the hormone and neurotransmitter oxytocin. Stories light up our brains. No wonder children don't ask for a bedtime fact, they ask for a bedtime story. Stories help us make order of a world bursting with uncertainty. The more fantastical, the better.

I was 11 years old when I learned about a fake moon landing. "*Cccclc-cchhhh*," my grandmother said, clicking her tongue as she drew the curtains. "*Cccclcchhhh*. The Americans didn't walk on the moon. Don't listen to their stories." We had finished saying evening prayers, our eyelids still warm from the special supplication whispered while looking at the moon, the *unwalked upon* moon. We had blown into our hands, pressed fingertips gently over our eyelids, and recited the moon prayer—a prayer for clarity and vision.

I rolled my turquoise velvet prayer mat into a long cheroot, tucked it beneath the settee, and looked at the yellow slice of light between the edges of the curtains my grandmother hadn't quite brought together. The moon. Its shape dictated our calendar, its sighting decided which day we would wear sparkly clothes and eat sweet Eid pastries.

My grandmother was a softly spoken woman with a round belly that she rested her hands on. She said little about the world, rarely commented on the small-town sagas that filled our days. This woman, born in a tiny village in India, living in a factory town in England, this sweet old woman of few words and even fewer opinions, was a conspiracy theorist?

We were a family of conspiracy theorists. After Sunday sermons at the mosque three streets away, my cousins and I would rush back to our home, form a half-moon around a black Sony cassette player and listen to Michael Jackson songs backward. "He's saying worship Satan!" my older cousin would claim, pressing the clunky stop button. "Listen! Michael Jackson is a devil worshiper!"

We studied the cover of his *Dangerous* album, drawing a line between the three monkey heads to form a pyramid, pointing to the red pentagram inside the pyramid, the couple—was it Adam and Eve?—trapped inside a glass orb. Signs of the Illuminati, we agreed, nodding our heads.

Even more entertaining than *Ghostbusters* and *The Neverending Story* were the tales of Aleister Crowley, the Knights of the Round Table, and the secrets behind the British Royal Family. One book we read and reread together told us that the Queen of England was a reptile in human form. A cassette tape we played over and over said Prince Charles was a shapeshifter who feasted on newborn babies. We lapped it up, our eyes wide with fear and wonder.

All of our childhoods we listened to stories about the monarchy and the British Empire. "Once upon a time, one in four humans on the planet was a subject of the British Empire," our parents' stories began.

That's wild, we said. *Sounds made up.*

On my cousin's blue and yellow bedroom wall was a map of the world in Gall-Peters projection, with every country the British had colonized colored in pink. There was our parents' birthplace, India. Pink. The birthplace of our grandparents, Burma. Pink. Entire swathes of continents ruled by an island nation small enough to fit into India eighteen times—at least according to its size before the British dragged a pencil across a map, sparked a genocide, and carved India into separate, warring nations.

Like stories of the Illuminati and shapeshifting monarchs, we reveled in the tales of a tiny island with the audacity to rule the planet. That map and our parents' stories were daily reminders that the absurd was possible; the cassette tape sermons evidence that the fantastical was more compelling than what the government purported to be the truth.

Besides, the official maps we studied in school were made up, the cassette tapes told us. Europeans had fudged the way we looked at the world and our home countries. Geert de Kremer, a sixteenth-century Flemish man, better known as Mercator, had drawn a map that shrank India and Africa and beefed up Europe. It was a conspiracy. But we had our stories. Stories that helped us band together against these travesties, to counter the narratives that made us small and them big. There was safety in numbers, and we found unity and relief in our collective beliefs.

So, years later, when I was 27, a newly qualified doctor working in east London, I was sympathetic to the pregnant young woman rolling her eyes, crossing her arms, and refusing my prescription. I was working in my local hospital, walking distance from my home, where many of my patients looked like me: young, brown, daughters of immigrants. They too had been raised on conspiracy theories about the government, the Queen, doctors.

"I don't want your antibiotics cuz they're poison," the young woman said, pulling the flimsy hospital sheet over her chest and kissing her teeth. Her sister-in-law had run a car over her feet during an argument, and an infection was setting in to her bloodied toes.

"I know you're worried about the baby," I said. "But this antibiotic is safe for both of you."

She didn't believe me. Medicines were multinational drug companies' way of controlling people of color, she said. They were tested on the poor and the voiceless to rake in profits for fat-cat CEOs. She wasn't the only person rejecting my interventions. Pregnant women refused ultrasounds believing the sonic waves would harm their baby's brain and heart. Fathers refused to vaccinate their toddlers.

A few years later when I was working as a public health doctor in the United States, one of the biggest tuberculosis outbreaks in the country's recent history spread through the city of Marion in Alabama. The TB rate in Marion was 100 times the national average and most of the people affected were Black Americans. Some Marion residents refused to get tested for the infection even when public health officials offered $20 as an incentive. The officials and doctors grumbled about the small numbers of Marion residents trickling in for blood tests and x-rays.

The doctors were ignoring history. A two-hour drive from Marion is Tuskegee, the site of a torturous, unethical medical experiment, conducted by government doctors on Black men from the 1930s to the 1970s. Even those residents of Marion who weren't alive when the experiment ended said that, because of those experiments, a distrust of medicine and doctors had been passed down through generations like an old family Bible.

These stories shouldn't be ignored. There is a bloody history packed into each aspirin pill: a story of Nazi concentration camps and Holocaust survivors.

There is a scandalous story behind the discovery of penicillin and its uses—and I'm not talking about the stories you learned in school about mold and petri dishes and Alexander Fleming.

These stories, and so many others like them that you will read in this book, are buried like dirty laundry considered too filthy to even try and wash. But their legacy lingers. We'd rather not wash our dirty linens in public because confronting the past raises difficult questions, like why *would* doctors inject bacteria into people's spines, and why *would* scientists not treat syphilis patients with medicine?

The true stories we bury sprout fake stories, like fungi blooming from dead tree trunks. There is sometimes an inkling of truth in a conspiracy theory, and these truths wrapped in history and suspicion can spread faster than microbes, infecting people with a deeper distrust of doctors and science. History is the kerosene that ignites conspiracy theories and fuels new hoaxes.

When I was 29, I joined the Epidemic Intelligence Service at the Centers for Disease Control and Prevention, a US government unit of medical sleuths who track contagions. Now that I was a federal disease detective chasing epidemics across the world, the conspiracy theories felt real again. I was sent to an American town where children were dying from a bacteria that could have been cured if they could afford a $12 antibiotic. In another American town, people were losing limbs and lives because they lacked clean running water and couldn't wash away a flesh-eating microbe. Outbreak after outbreak, I was confronted with strange pathogens and stranger human behaviors and beliefs. These experiences convinced me that working as a public health doctor was not enough to improve public health. I had to train as an expert storyteller, master the art of crafting stories, and combine narrative with medicine to make people care.

In the summer of 2014, as Ebola was raging in West Africa, I unpacked boxes in my new home in north Texas and questioned my latest career decision. I had left my job as a disease detective at the CDC, graduated from journalism school, and was preparing for my first job as a newspaper reporter at the *Dallas Morning News*. While I was making a home in the suburbs of Dallas, my disease detective friends were zipping up Tyvek suits and climbing into Ebola treatment units in Guinea, Liberia, and Sierra Leone. I fluffed pillows and swallowed guilt.

And then Ebola arrived in Dallas. All of a sudden north Texas was ground zero for a virus named after a river in central Africa. My worlds collided and I stepped into the role of public health translator, debunker of myths about viruses and how they spread, and according to my editor in chief, the voice of calm and reason amid hysterical news reports.

It was a friend at the CDC who told me the story about the mother in Texas demanding an Ebola vaccine while refusing the flu shot. We chuckled about the mother's request, but then we stopped and looked at each other nervously. In the scheme of things that keep public health doctors awake at night, flu is near top of the list. That virus kills tens of thousands of Americans each year and sickens millions. Eventually, my friend was deployed to Sierra Leone to help with the Ebola outbreak response and I was sent to Liberia to report on the epidemic for *Scientific American*. In Liberia, some people told me the virus had been spread either maliciously by the US government or accidentally, in an experiment gone awry, by Tulane University scientists. It seemed that news about the outbreak, some of it accurate, some of it untrue, spread faster than the infection.

When I returned home to Texas, readers of my newspaper flooded my inbox with angry emails: "Y'all know Ebola is airborne but y'all won't admit it!" And: "Illegals are bringing Ebola from Mexico. Shut down the border!!!" We were the purveyors of truth, but nobody was buying our message.

Medical myths and pseudoscience converged to cause hysteria. Some Texas schools closed for a thorough cleaning even though not a single person with Ebola had been anywhere near the buildings. The repercussions reverberated beyond Texas. A bridal store in Ohio went out of business when a Dallas nurse, who was later diagnosed with Ebola, was found to have visited the boutique days before she was contagious. West Africans living in north Texas were turned away from their jobs by employers who believed they could be contagious.

Those reactions were dangerous, ill-informed, and expensive to the taxpayer. Other conspiracy theories cost people their lives. Beliefs that traditional medicines could cure Ebola led to flare-ups of the virus in places where the epidemic was previously under control.

It's easy to mock some beliefs as antiscience and stupid, but at some point in our lives, probably all of us are that mother in the Texas pediatrician's office worrying more about the absurd danger than the quotidian one. We worry about dying in a plane crash more than we think about dying in a car. We worry about exotic infections more than we worry about that reliable killer, flu. Humans are notoriously poor at evaluating risks, study after study has proven so. Now, aided by social media and a twenty-four-hour news cycle, fear and misinformation spread fast and fuel our panic and poor decisions.

Nowadays I track the spread of microbes and misinformation, a combination named misinfodemics by experts Nat Gyenes and An Xiao Mina. I try not to judge the false health news that spreads. Raised on conspiracy theories, I understand why a patient might refuse medications, say chemtrails are poison, or shun vaccines, even as I bristle at the public health implications of these beliefs and behaviors.

Public health officials try to counter false health news with "facts," but this book questions the very idea of facts and the experiments, methods, and systems through which so-called facts are established. Whatever you think of facts, facts alone are not convincing. Stories are what we remember. This book dissects those stories, from medical myths about vaccines and chemtrails, to conspiracy theories about nefarious governments and unscrupulous scientists. Each chapter explores where the stories come from and why they stick in our minds. Throughout the book, whether talking about baby powder and ovarian cancer, or diet pills and kidney failure, we return to these three questions: why do we believe what we believe, why don't facts extinguish falsehoods, and what is a fact, anyway?

01

Do the flat tummy detox teas touted by Instagram celebrities actually work?

O ne morning, I reached for my bottle of birth control pills, swallowed one with a gulp of tea, and realized I had accidentally poisoned myself. Instead of a mix of progesterone and estrogen, I had downed my dog's thyroid pill. The medicine for her underactive gland was a dose of thyroid hormone many times higher than what I would prescribe for a human. I did what any rational person with a medical degree would do. I freaked out.

A series of bad decisions had led to the accidental poisoning. First, I had decanted my pills from their packaging, which was specially designed to help busy women take the right pill on the right day. Then, I had packed the pills into an empty bottle of antihistamines I had run through during my summer bout of hay fever. I had placed this mislabeled antihistamine bottle of birth control medicine next to Lily's too-high-dosage-for-a-human thyroid tablets so we could both be good girls and take our pills on time in the morning.

What could possibly go wrong?

I called an emergency room doctor–friend who had an idea. On his suggestion, I ran to the drugstore and cleaned them out of "detox" tablets. Hunched over my kitchen countertop, I split open 100 neon pink gelatin capsules (why were they pink?, I wondered later when I cleaned up the empty shells), shook the charcoal powder into a glass, mixed it with water to make a thick sludge and swallowed with as much enthusiasm as I could muster. My kitchen and my lily-white dog were blanketed in a fine layer of black charcoal dust.

Activated charcoal stops poison from being absorbed by the gut. The idea is to stop the poison ending up in your bloodstream, and it can work if you take the activated charcoal within an hour of poisoning.

I don't recommend what I did (don't take your dog's meds, don't take charcoal at home—if you're worried enough to take charcoal, you should get it from an ER doctor, who will pour it out of a bottle like a normal person and not empty 100 capsules in a kitchen). But I was intrigued that charcoal was sold in such small doses in a drugstore. My ER doctor–friend who I had called in a panic, knew it would be on sale there. "They sell charcoal because people take it to quote unquote detox," he had said.

But in 250 milligram doses, charcoal powder, which probably isn't the activated version used in the ER anyway, doesn't really do anything. Claims that it cures bad breath and that two capsules will absorb toxins from a diet of sodas and fried chicken are false promises.

Much of what we have been taught about nutrition is being debunked these days. A plate half full of starches such as rice, pasta, or potatoes is now considered unhealthy. Fat was the demon in the eighties, but sugar—a white powder considered as addictive as cocaine, peddled by an industry that paid scientists to tell us fat was more harmful than sugar—is being outed as the real evil.

Nutrition science has left our questions unanswered or answered them with half-truths. And where there are unanswered questions, there are scammers, snake oil salesmen and women who ply us with promises of a toned tummy.

Diet fads aren't new; even detox teas have been around for decades, but they are being sold to us in a different way. And the detox industry is big business. There are juice cleanses, cheese cleanses, detox teas and tinctures, and your favorite celebrities can be seen on Instagram pouting while holding any one of these scams. Some are paid tens of thousands of dollars to pose fish-faced and take selfies with "fit teas" and "flat tummy teas." They are part of the multimillion-dollar industry that promises to quickly tighten and tone while you lay on your couch and hand over your credit card.

These quick fixes don't work. They do drain you of some water and make you poop for days, both of which make you weigh less when you stand on a scale. But this is weight that is quickly regained when you stop taking the supplements.

And while detoxes and cleanses won't fix you, they could kill you. In 2017 a 60-year-old woman in Philadelphia died after a cleanse involving detox tea. She had been drinking Yogi DeTox tea three times a day for two weeks before she went to the doctor feeling weak and lethargic. Her skin and eyes had turned yellow and she was admitted to the hospital. Nine days into her admission she became disoriented and confused. Her liver was failing. A biopsy revealed black, dying liver tissue.

On day fifteen she had to be intubated. She died on day seventeen.

The doctors looked at the list of nineteen ingredients in the detox tea and found six that were known to cause liver injury, among them: gardenia fruit, rhubarb root, juniper berry, cinnamon bark, and skullcap root.

Some ingredients in the tea were said to protect the liver, but those claims were based on experiments in mice, the researchers said. They warned that "herbal products are contaminated with other toxins or added adulterants that are not advertised on the packaging," which could lead to a "cluster effect," where more than one toxic ingredient bombards the liver until it can't cope, shuts down, and dies. It didn't help that the woman drank three glasses of wine a night, the doctors said. This combination of wine and harmless-sounding but toxic "cleansing" herbs was the likely cause of her death.

Detox teas and cleanses can also land you on the maternity ward. One of the ingredients in many detox products is senna, a medicine used to treat constipation. Senna irritates the bowel so that it contracts, water enters the intestines, and you poop watery diarrhea. It's the medicine used in hospitals to clean out the bowel before endoscopy and bowel surgery.

Dumping a pound of feces will make you lighter on the weighing scale, but it can also make you poop out your birth control, making it less effective and an unplanned pregnancy more likely.

Senna is an herb approved by the Food and Drug Administration for short-term use to treat constipation; that's why you might see the labels "natural" or "clinically proven" on some detox and cleanse products. Be wary. Some herbs at particular doses can be deadly.

Senna is available without a prescription, but it's intended for short-term use and not as a weight loss tool. Besides causing severe abdominal cramps and dehydration, taken in high doses or for longer than two weeks, senna can cause dependence as well as muscle weakness, liver damage, and heart disorders.

Caffeine is another additive in some weight loss and "flat tummy" products, especially those advertised for use during the day. Caffeine is a diuretic, meaning it makes you pee, and gives you a kick of energy. Other diuretics are also included in products, but losing water weight is not a long-term weight loss solution. The weight will creep back on as soon as you stop taking a diuretic.

One company, Flat Tummy Co., started off selling its senna-laced tea and progressed to lollipops that were supposed to make you eat less. The company used inspirational mantras as part of its social media strategy, even quotes from Nelson Mandela.

Upset employees spoke to journalists in 2018 on the condition of anonymity and described how the company used celebrities and social media influencers to skyrocket sales. Staff were asked to contact hundreds of influencers each, ideally those with at least 100,000 Instagram followers. They were paid from $25 dollars per post up to tens of thousands of dollars depending on their stardom. "We never expected them to actually use the tea," one former employee told the *Guardian*. "It just had to look like it."

Describing how they picked women, one employee said, "You don't want someone who already has a six pack. You want a mum who is on her fit journey trying to lose weight after having kids." Another former employee told the *Guardian*, "If someone is a little bit bigger, they get a higher rating than if someone's skinny. No one is going to listen to a skinny white girl say that she bought this tea and it's great."

"Models were downgraded if they were too 'slutty' on the assumption that their followers would be mostly male," the article said.

But the company and others like it were onto something with their use of influencers. The celeb effect is real. When Angelina Jolie announced in the op-ed pages of the *New York Times* in 2013 that she had had a double mastectomy because of a family history of breast cancer and a genetic test result that showed she carried the *BRCA1* gene mutation with a higher risk for breast cancer, it sparked a massive rise in women worried about cancer. Clinics were inundated with women asking to be screened for genetic mutations.

There was a 64 percent uptick in breast cancer genetic testing in the two weeks after Angelina Jolie's announcement, said Harvard researchers who looked through records of more than 9 million American women ages 18 to 64. There was no spike during the same time period the previous year.

The "Angelina Jolie effect" went global. Across the United Kingdom, Australia, United States, Canada, and Austria, there was an overall 285 percent increase in referrals for breast and ovarian cancer and an 80 percent increase in *BRCA* gene testing, according to scientists at the University of Siena in Italy. The upticks in referrals didn't correspond with a rise in mastectomies or actual diagnoses of breast cancer.

"Our findings underscore celebrity endorsements as a powerful influence on health-related behaviors, but they also show that such endorsements do not necessarily target those most at risk for developing a disease," said Sunita Desai, a Harvard researcher.

The Angelina Jolie effect was one of the first times scientists studied the impact of celebrities on our medical decision making. Their influence on the way we dress and eat has already been well documented.

When it comes to potentially harmful supplements, we're shown the glamorous aftereffects by people paid to pose with products they are often not taking themselves. In the case of detox teas and so-called cleanses, photos of hospital visits for dehydration, kidney failure, liver damage, heart palpitations, and nonstop diarrhea don't end up on Instagram with the tags #flattummyteascam or #flattummyteacantstoppooping. It's not as sexy to pout for the camera and say a balanced diet and exercise are the best ways to lose fat and gain muscle, so don't expect your favorite celebrity to say that anytime soon. But keep in mind that behind the filters and the pouts, there are multimillion-dollar companies paying influencers to make false claims. The detox and cleanse industries are a dangerous scam.

02

Should you eat your baby's placenta?

I n the fall of September 2016 an Oregon baby fell sick soon after it was born. Feverish and struggling to breathe, the baby was taken to the hospital, where it was admitted to the neonatal intensive care unit. Doctors inserted a needle into the baby's back to test the fluid around its spinal cord and drew blood to check for bugs. They found the bacteria Group B Streptococcus in the baby's bloodstream.

Doctors were puzzled. The mother had been tested for this bacterium during pregnancy—women in the United States are checked for Group B Streptococcus around the thirty-fifth week of pregnancy with a sterile swab inserted into the vagina. This mother had tested negative.

The doctors gave the baby antibiotics and sent the family home, but after only a few days the baby was back in the hospital. This time the mother told the medical team about a supplement she was taking: every day since giving birth she had swallowed two pills a few times a day. The pills were gelatin capsules containing one of her organs. A company had freeze-dried her placenta, ground it finely, and packed it into pills.

The placenta is a dark red fetal organ about two inches thick, smooth and slippery on top and rough on the bottom. It grows alongside the baby during pregnancy. It usually weighs about a pound and has a strange metallic smell and is considered biohazardous waste that hospitals usually incinerate. Sometimes women ask to take the placenta home so they can bury it for cultural or religious reasons.

For years, celebrities and specialist companies have promoted the so-called benefits of swallowing the placenta, and some experts say that thousands of women in the United States are frying their placenta with onions or blending the organ in smoothies. Some eat it raw (it tastes a bit like liver and other organ meats, I'm told), some freeze-dry the organ and stuff it into gelatin capsules, like the mother in Oregon. If you look online, you'll find recipes for placenta lasagna and a placenta roast. There are also placenta tacos and, in case you have a sweet tooth, placenta truffles.

Some celebrities swear by it. Kim Kardashian claimed that swallowing her placenta speeded up her postpartum recovery and kept her looking young. She advised her pregnant sister to line up a "placenta person" who would drop by the delivery suite, whisk the placenta away, and bring it back in pill form. Actress January Jones claimed that eating her placenta helped her fight postpartum depression. Some say it helps them breast-feed, but there is no evidence to support these claims. In fact, one of the hormones in the placenta is estrogen, which can actually make it more difficult to produce breast milk.

Researchers at the University of Nevada, Las Vegas, checked out these claims by studying 23,000 births. One in three women in their study ate her baby's placenta, but none, the researchers said, seemed to pass on the infection to their baby. They learned that women with anxiety and depression were more likely to eat the placenta, with most of them saying they were trying to prevent postpartum depression.

In another study researchers checked out the claims made by celebs by giving some women placenta pills and others placebo pills. The claim that eating your placenta keeps away the baby blues are unfounded, they said, and potentially harmful. A mother relying on placenta pills to keep the postnatal depression away might forego treatments that are proven to work.

Placenta-eating proponents say it makes sense to eat the organ because it's laden with blood and hormones. But it can also be full of infection. Sometimes this is obvious from the way the placenta looks or if it stinks, but other times the bugs are concealed within the placenta and it's hard to tell that bacteria are lurking inside.

Placenta eaters point to animals, saying new mothers should eat their placentas because monkeys do. But for wild animals, the practice is probably a way to clean up and get rid of the smell of blood, which can attract predators.

In the case of the Oregon mother, it's likely she didn't suffer any symptoms herself from eating the bacteria-laced placenta pills. Her breast milk tested negative for the infection, but the same kind of Group B Streptococcus found in her placenta pills was found swimming inside the baby's blood. In fact, when scientists from the Centers for Disease Control and Prevention investigated, they ran tests to compare the bacteria in the placenta pills with the bacteria in blood samples taken from the baby when it was in the hospital, twice.

They used a test called whole genome sequencing, which compares the genes of bacteria, and found no genetic differences between the strains. Another test, pulsed-field gel electrophoresis, couldn't distinguish between the bacteria in the placental pills and the bacteria inside the baby, either.

The mother had given her placenta to a company that freeze-dries the organs, grinds them into powder, and turns them into gelatin capsules. Luckily, the mother told her doctors about the placenta pills, information that helped the CDC investigate the illness. The baby was treated with antibiotics for close to a month and survived the infection.

But if she hadn't shared that information or if the bacterial infection wasn't treated, it could have killed the baby. Group B Streptococcus causes lung, brain, and blood infections in newborns as well as infections of the bones and joints. About one in four pregnant women carries the bacteria in her vagina or rectum. That's why the CDC recommends testing all pregnant women between thirty-five to thirty-seven weeks of pregnancy. If the bacteria are found inside the vagina, the woman is treated with antibiotics during labor to stop the bug being passed to the baby.

The placenta-eating trend offers a new way for newborns to pick up the bacteria. Be wary of companies and celebrities peddling placentas as a health miracle. The placenta is a fetal organ designed to help the baby receive oxygen inside the womb. It can be riddled with feces, inflammatory cells, and bacteria, and eating it could harm your baby.

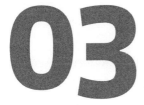

Do vaccines cause autism?

The biggest outbreak of measles to hit the midwestern state of Minnesota in almost thirty years spread across the city of Minneapolis in the spring of 2017. Nearly eighty people were sickened with the virus, many hospitalized with fevers and problems breathing, and most of the sick were children, some as young as a year old.

By June 2017, there were more people sick with measles in Minnesota than in the entire United States the previous year. Eight out of ten of the children infected in the Minnesota measles outbreak were Somali-American children who were unvaccinated. For almost a decade, their parents had been carefully targeted by groups who told them vaccines were dangerous and cause autism.

They were lied to. Vaccines save lives and thousands of studies, some of them tracking the health of a million children, have proven childhood vaccines for diseases such as measles, mumps, and whooping cough are safe. But since a fraudulent study was published in the *Lancet* medical journal in 1998 claiming that vaccines cause autism, an antivaccine movement has been spreading across the world.

The now-retracted *Lancet* paper was written by a British doctor, Andrew Wakefield, who experimented on twelve children with signs of autism. Wakefield did spinal taps and colonoscopies on the children, took their blood at a kid's birthday party, and fudged what parents told him about their children's symptoms to fit his hypothesis that the measles, mumps, and rubella, or MMR, vaccine was dangerous.

He said that some of the kids developed signs of autism after getting the MMR shot even though parents said their kids had the symptoms before. A medical review board said Wakefield treated the kids like guinea pigs by doing unnecessary, invasive medical tests, including putting scopes up their backsides.

Why would a researcher make stuff up?

In 1996, Wakefield was put on payroll by a lawyer who wanted to sue the MMR vaccine maker. The lawyer needed evidence that the vaccine caused harm, so he paid Wakefield around half a million pounds (approximately $700,000) and funded his unethical "study."

Brian Deer, a British journalist, unearthed Wakefield's lies and cash flow by interviewing parents of the children whom Wakefield experimented on and by following the money trail. Wakefield didn't tell the medical journal about this conflict of interest, and he denies Deer's claims.

After the results of his fraudulent study were published in the *Lancet* in 1998, Wakefield said something interesting at a press conference. It hinted at a potential motive. Even though his study results didn't show it, he suggested that individual vaccines for measles, mumps, and rubella could be safer than one combined vaccine. Wakefield was keeping another secret. What he didn't disclose was that nine months before that press conference he had filed a patent for a single-dose measles vaccine. He stood to profit from his made-up science.

Wakefield lost his UK medical license in 2010, the same year the *Lancet* retracted his fraudulent study—yes, it took the now not-so-esteemed journal twelve years to retract the study that had caused so much harm. Vaccination rates in the United Kingdom and United States had decreased, and outbreaks of vaccine-preventable diseases such as measles and whooping cough had risen. Public health experts blame Wakefield and his followers.

Wakefield moved to Texas. He doubled down on his false "vaccines cause autism" rhetoric, despite solid scientific proof that there is no link between vaccines and autism. In the United States Wakefield has the ear of President Donald Trump and Hollywood celebrities such as Jim Carrey, and he is the icon for a growing antivaccine movement.

A few years before the Minnesota measles outbreak, Wakefield made repeat visits to Minneapolis. (During one 2011 visit where he addressed community members, Wakefield had armed guards preventing journalists and actual doctors from entering the room to hear what he had to say.)

He had been invited by Minnesota's Somali community, who were worried about what they perceived to be a high rate of autism diagnoses in Somali children. A small survey by the Minnesota Department of Health in 2008 found that more Somali children in Minneapolis were enrolled in special education autism programs, compared to Black non-Somali, Hispanic, and white kids. But a 2013 study found Somali children were about as likely as white children to be diagnosed with autism, according to researchers at the University of Minnesota.

Around the same time as the first autism study, nine years before the measles outbreak hit Minneapolis, concerned Somali parents were looking for answers to their questions about autism and intellectual disabilities in their community.

Groups such as the Organic Consumers Association, an antivaccine organization, were invited to talk to the community and answer questions. They shared their antivaccine beliefs. Vaccination rates in the Somali community began to drop.

The impact was staggering. Rates of MMR vaccination among Somali children born in the United States used to be higher compared to kids of other races and ethnicities in Minnesota. That changed drastically in 2014. The MMR vaccination rate in Somali children dropped from 92 percent in 2004 to 42 percent a decade later.

That's a frighteningly high proportion of unvaccinated kids. One in ten kids who has measles suffers with lifelong hearing loss. For every 1,000 kids with measles, one will suffer swelling of the brain resulting in seizures and learning disabilities, and one or two will die. And many years after a child is thought to have made a full recovery from measles, a disease called subacute sclerosing panencephalitis, or SSPE, can strike. The brain swells against the skull, the child suffers mood swings, depression, and dementia, and dies within two years of being diagnosed with SSPE.

In 2016 it was discovered that SSPE is more common than previously thought. Children who get measles before the age of 1 have a 1 in 609 chance of developing SSPE. For kids infected with measles before the age of 5, the risk is 1 in 1,387. Still, some who refuse to believe that vaccines are life-saving describe measles as a "mild disease."

Vaccines are more than a personal decision: getting vaccinated is a civic duty. To protect a community from the terrors of measles, around 93 percent of people in the community need to be vaccinated. When the vaccination rate falls below that level, everyone is at risk of infection, especially children who are too young to be vaccinated and people who are sick with cancer or other illnesses.

Before Minnesota's biggest measles epidemic in thirty years, Andrew Wakefield visited the Somali community more than once to share his antivaccine message. "The Somalis had decided themselves that they were particularly concerned. I was responding to that," he told the *Washington Post*. About the state's measles outbreak, he said, "I don't feel responsible at all."

Suaado Salah, a 26-year-old mother who moved to Minnesota from Somalia, had a 3-year-old son and an 18-month-old daughter who were both infected with measles during the 2017 epidemic. "I thought: 'I'm in America. I thought I'm in a safe place and my kids will never get sick in that disease,'" she told the *Washington Post*. Salah had been sick with measles herself when she was a girl in Somalia. Her 3-year-old sister had died from measles.

In the wake of the epidemic, the Centers for Disease Control and Prevention studied vaccination rates in Minnesota. "Overall, children with at least one foreign-born parent were 25 percent less likely to be current on their vaccinations at 36 months than were children born to two U.S.-born parents, after adjusting for maternal race, age, and educational attainment," the researchers said.

If both parents or even one parent was born outside the United States, the child was more likely not to be "up-to-date on vaccinations at ages 2, 6, and 18 months, and not to be caught up by age 36 months," the study found.

Vaccination rates were different for children, depending on where their parents were from. Around eight out of ten children whose mothers were from the

Caribbean or Central and South America were vaccinated. Fewer than five out of ten kids whose mothers were from Somalia were vaccinated.

That difference could stem from the Somali community's worries about autism, a concern that antivaccine groups had stepped in to address in a way the public health department had not. Sure, science explains that vaccines don't cause autism, wrote the *Washington Post's* Lena Sun. But for many parents in the Somali community, the feeling was "science should be able to say what *does.*"

Measles was eliminated from the United States in 2000. Now, thanks to Wakefield and his antivaccine movement, the virus is back with a vengeance. Whooping cough, rubella, mumps—arcane infections of our grandparents' generations—are making a comeback. After I investigated an outbreak of whooping cough in Phoenix, Arizona, in 2011, I presented the findings at the CDC's annual Epidemic Intelligence Service conference the next year. An older man in the audience stood up after my talk to share a memory. He said his baby brother had died of whooping cough in the 1950s. He described how a trip to the cinema back then was punctuated with the throaty *whooooop* of children infected with the bacteria. "We have vaccines now," he said. "And it's anathema to me that people are refusing them."

The outbreak of whooping cough I investigated as a disease detective occurred in a neonatal intensive care unit, home to arguably the hospital's most precious, most fragile residents. These preemies with their paper-thin translucent skin, were coughing so hard they were turning blue. One newborn infected in the outbreak had recently had open heart surgery. I was worried he would die from whooping cough.

When I traced the likely source of the infection, I wanted to throw my laptop out of the window. It turned out that some of the nurses, respiratory therapists, and other health care workers caring for the babies were unvaccinated and—worse still—had carried on working in the neonatal intensive care unit while they were coughing and spluttering with whooping cough.

"Why would you come to work *in the NICU* when you have whooping cough and are coughing over preemies?" I asked them, feeling extremely frustrated and yes, furious, but trying to be open-minded. "Sick time is lumped together with personal time," I was told. There was an incentive to continue working through sickness. In a medical journal article, I blamed the outbreak on the hospital system's dangerous sick-leave policy. "Do an economic analysis," my boss, Dr. Rebecca Sunenshine told me. "Calculate how much this outbreak cost the hospital." She said it was the only way of making the hospital executives care. So I did. The total cost was $97,745 and, of course, the incalculable cost of nearly losing five babies. It didn't change anything.

Shouldn't health care workers have to be vaccinated to care for the already sick and vulnerable? Two patients died and twenty-five were sickened with flu in Memorial Sloan Kettering Cancer Center in New York in 1998. Only 12 percent of health care workers in the bone marrow unit where the deaths occurred had been vaccinated against the flu. In another fatal flu outbreak, one baby died and nineteen were sickened in a neonatal intensive care unit in Canada. Only 15 percent of health care workers were vaccinated.

Flu vaccines are mandatory for people working in hospitals in some regions such as Alameda County in northern California. In other places, health care workers—yes, I know this sounds counterintuitive—have revolted against mandatory vaccinations. In 2013, the National Union of Nurses and Hospital Employees stalled a University of New Mexico mandatory vaccine policy. And when New York State mandated flu vaccinations for health care workers in 2009, unions obtained a court injunction that stopped the mandate. In 2013, New York responded by requiring unvaccinated health care workers to wear masks during flu season.

In a 2018 study of 359 nurses in the northeastern United States, only two out of three nurses agreed that the flu vaccine is safe. Earlier surveys of nurses who refused the flu vaccine found some who believed the vaccine could make them sick. This is worrying, given that patients look to health care workers for guidance when making personal decisions about vaccines.

The year before I investigated the outbreak of whooping cough in the NICU, there were 27,550 cases of whooping cough in the United States, almost triple the number seen in 2007. That number rose to more than 48,000 in 2012. That year twenty Americans died from whooping cough, sixteen of them younger than a year old.

The same antivaccine sentiment is spreading across the world. Romania, Italy, and Brazil have seen outbreaks of diseases that could be prevented with vaccines.

Some communities have valid reasons for not believing health claims made by governments, drug companies, and scientists. Antivaccine groups know this and exploit it. Antivaccine groups have been working with the Nation of Islam, a Black American religious organization, to lie to Black parents and tell them all vaccines are poisons. Some call the antivaccine propaganda sharers "the white supporters of Minister Louis Farrakhan," the leader of the Nation of Islam. Which is interesting, given that Farrakhan refers to white people as the devil.

But Farrakhan makes a valid point when he references recent medical history and tells his congregation to beware the medical establishment. As recently as 1973, Black men living in Alabama were left to suffer with syphilis as part of a government study run by the US Public Health Service. The Tuskegee Study of Untreated Syphilis in the Negro Male ran from 1932 to 1973, during which time a cure for syphilis—penicillin—was discovered. But the Black men were denied penicillin by government doctors. Instead, the untreated men infected their wives and unborn babies with the bacteria, which can cause irreversible organ damage. All the while, government doctors documented their suffering. Farrakhan draws on this history to spread disinformation about vaccines, which save lives.

More recently there have been studies showing that white American doctors and medical students harbor magical beliefs about Black bodies. Half the white medical students and residents in a 2016 University of Virginia study believed such absurdities as "blacks age more slowly than whites; their nerve endings are less sensitive than whites'; their blood coagulates more quickly than whites'; their skin is thicker than whites'." Those who believed that Black bodies are different from white bodies were "more likely to report lower pain ratings for the black vs. white patient, and were less accurate in their treatment recommendations for the black vs. white patient."

Farrakhan's congregation has reason to be wary when he warns, "They are vaccinating our black babies." Videos of his preaching uploaded to YouTube show him telling parents to refuse one of the first injections given to babies. But that injection is not a vaccine. It's a shot of vitamin K given to newborns. We are born with a vitamin K deficiency and only start making the vitamin in our gut later in childhood. The vitamin is crucial to proper clotting of blood. Without the vitamin K injection, babies can suffer brain and intestine hemorrhages that can kill them. That's why an intramuscular vitamin K shot has been recommended in the United States since 1961.

But half the pediatricians in a 2017 survey in the United States said that over a five-year period, they had witnessed an increase in parents refusing the vitamin K injection for their newborns. Around one in ten said they dealt with a parent refusing the injection on a weekly basis; one in three said it was a monthly occurrence. The risk for babies developing vitamin K deficiency bleeding (VKDB) is more than eighty times higher for babies who do not get the injection. For every five babies with VKDB, one will die from it.

While antivaccine (and even anti–vitamin K injection) groups are targeting those vulnerable to disinformation, including Black communities such as Minnesota's Somali population and members of the Nation of Islam, the majority of Americans who refuse vaccines are white and educated. Parents who reject or plan to reject the vitamin K injection are mostly white, college-educated, and over the age of 30, keeping with the demographic trend for parents who refuse to vaccinate their kids.

There are different reasons for vaccine refusal in different communities, and antivaccine groups are targeting communities based on preexisting beliefs. Armed with conspiracy theories about corruption in the CDC and a secret government plan to annihilate Black babies, the antivaccine movement concocts and disseminates targeted stories.

Even after the Institute of Medicine analyzed 1,000 studies to conclude that the MMR vaccine is safe, and Danish researchers followed more than half a million kids to come to the same conclusion: some parents choose not to vaccinate their children. Some health care workers choose not to get vaccinated and cough all over their patients instead.

The antivaccine horror story will not be conquered with facts alone. In some studies where researchers used facts about mumps and measles, parents who didn't like vaccines to begin with actually doubled down on their antivaccine sentiment.

Wakefield's experiments have been called the biggest fraud in medical history. Combined with a sordid history of exploitation and experimentation of the most vulnerable people, antivaxxers have whipped up a perfect storm of conditions to spread their deadly message. Vaccines save lives. We have to do better at sharing that message.

04

Can autism be cured?

Industrial bleach, clay powder, parasitic worms. These are some of the "treatments" being offered to children with autism by medical providers promising to "cure" their autism.

One in sixty-eight children in the United States is diagnosed with autism spectrum disorder (ASD) by age 8, according to the Centers for Disease Control and Prevention. Autism is a neurodevelopmental disorder characterized by repetitive behavior, communication problems, and difficulty engaging in social interactions and forming relationships.

There is no cure for autism, but a growing number of medical providers are preying on parents of autistic children. These charlatans, ranging from doctors to chiropractors to naturopaths, claim autism is caused by heavy metal poisoning, digestive issues, or metabolic problems that can be treated with expensive, unproven, and sometimes dangerous practices, including infection with parasites.

Their websites claim that interventions such as hyperbaric oxygen therapy have been "clinically demonstrated to provide symptomatic relief and increase quality of life for patients suffering from several chronic and acute conditions."

The Food and Drug Administration warns against using products that claim to reverse autism. Children have died after receiving the "autism reversal" medicine known as Miracle Mineral Solution (MMS), which is actually chloride dioxide, another name for industrial bleach.

One-third to 43 percent of families in the United States pay for these alternative treatments for children with autism, according to some studies. The peddlers of fake cures know exactly what they are doing. They enlist high-profile speakers and celebrities to speak at their conventions. An autism convention in Dallas in 2016, the Autism Education Summit, was hosted by Generation Rescue, an organization co-founded by antivaccine advocate Jenny McCarthy, who has a son with autism. McCarthy was joined by a Texas district attorney who also claims vaccines cause autism.

The event featured a medical professional who was disciplined for mistreating children and two doctors facing lawsuits for using dangerous treatments, which they claim reverse autism. Anjum Usman and Daniel Rossignol were sued in Chicago by the parent of a 7-year-old boy with autism. The boy's father, James Coman, said the doctors harmed his son using "dangerous and unnecessary experimental treatments."

Rossignol and Usman prescribed intravenous chelation treatments designed to rid the body of heavy metals. Chelation treatment is approved only for treating conditions such as lead poisoning and iron overload and even then, side effects can include high blood pressure, abnormal heart rhythms, and low calcium, which can cause the heart to stop. Rossignol prescribed the treatments over the phone without ever seeing the 7-year-old, the lawsuit said.

Studies have found that chelation does not cure autism and can be dangerous when used to treat the condition. In a study by researchers at Cornell University, rats with no lead exposure treated with a chelator sometimes given to children with autism suffered long-term impairment of emotional regulation and brain function.

A 5-year-old boy died in Pennsylvania in 2005 during his third session of chelation treatment. He was treated by Dr. Roy Kerry, who believed the boy's autism was caused by heavy metal poisoning. An autopsy showed the child's death was caused by brain injury and heart damage due to a drop in calcium levels. Kerry voluntarily surrendered his medical license in 2008. Usman and Rossignol are part of a group called Defeat Autism Now!, which promotes so-called autism treatments that are discredited and disproved by science. Usman's medical license has been put on probation.

Peddlers of fake cures point to the rise in autism diagnoses in the United States to back up their false theories that autism is caused by exposure to heavy metals or certain foods.

Autism is more common in the United States today than it was in the 1980s, and the number is steadily rising. One in fifty-nine kids was diagnosed with ASD in 2014, compared to one in sixty-eight in 2012. A study published in 2015 found that a broader definition of autism could explain why more children are diagnosed with the disorder. While researchers cannot pinpoint the cause of autism, many agree that a number of factors including genes and environmental exposures probably interact and play a role in the development of the condition.

Unanswered questions about the rise in diagnoses offered a platform for antivaccine groups to answer those queries with their own misinformed opinions. "A number of these speakers are opportunists and predators who prey on the fears and the desperation of parents who have kids with autism," said Dr. Peter Hotez, a pediatrician at Baylor College of Medicine in Houston whose daughter has autism. Hotez wrote a book, *Vaccines Did Not Cause Rachel's Autism,* sharing his experiences as an autism father and vaccine researcher. "I understand how desperate and hopeless a parent can feel having a child with autism and it doesn't get better with age because now we're dealing with a young adult with autism."

Fiona O'Leary, an autism rights advocate from Ireland who is on the autism spectrum, said autism summits like the one in Dallas in 2016 pretend to be about people living with autism while serving only to promote dangerous myths and medicines. "What we need to be doing is supporting people with autism and listening to them but we're not invited because they don't want to hear from us," said O'Leary, who has two children with autism. She cites the summit's lack of autistic speakers as evidence that the words and experiences of those living with the condition are not important to the organizers.

O'Leary founded a nonprofit in Ireland, Autistic Rights Together, that campaigns for better regulation of treatments that purport to reverse autism. "We are vulnerable," she said. "Parents are vulnerable, many don't have support and they're being fed misinformation by charities like Generation Rescue."

O'Leary said she was threatened by a doctor who prescribes the industrial bleach "medicine" known as the Miracle Mineral Solution when she spoke about the dangers of the treatment. "They don't care about people with autism," she said. "They threaten people with autism who dare to speak up."

Besides promoting useless and sometimes dangerous treatments, doctors prey on parents of children with autism by using meaningless diagnostic tests. To "prove" to parents that their child has heavy metal poisoning, urine is tested for metals after the child is given a chelation treatment. The problem with these tests is that the healthy human body contains trace amounts of metals and there's no standard reference range for the amount of these elements a person excretes in urine after chelation treatment.

But labs that collude with quack doctors send back alarming results that appear to show high levels of metal in the child's urine. These are contrasted with a so-called reference range taken from a person who has not been given chelation treatment.

The American College of Medical Toxicology has said chelation treatment does not improve symptoms of autism and that " 'provoked' or 'challenge' tests of urine are not reliable means to diagnose metal poisoning and have been associated with harm."

The onus is on families to protect themselves from health care workers and businesspeople peddling expensive treatments and false hope. While the FDA is cracking down on fraudulent treatments, the agency does not keep up with the myriad miracle cures that claim to reverse autism.

Here are some of the fake autism reversal treatments to watch out for.

Hyperbaric oxygen therapy involves inhaling oxygen inside a pressurized chamber. It is approved by the FDA for treating decompression sickness in scuba divers but is not approved for treating autism. One flawed study claimed the treatment is effective, while numerous studies have shown it does not treat autism.

Clay bath powders are said to detoxify the body by drawing out heavy metals and chemical toxins. The FDA has investigated manufacturers claiming these clay baths offer "dramatic improvement" for symptoms of autism. A clay bath powder will not change the brain of a child with ASD.

Miracle Mineral Solution is bleach, and it's really not wise to make children drink bleach (I never thought I'd have to say that). Its sellers would like you to believe them when they tell you on their website that MMS is "the answer to AIDS, hepatitis A, B and C, malaria, herpes, TB, most cancer and many more of mankind's worst diseases." The FDA has received reports of people who have suffered severe vomiting and severely low blood pressure after drinking this solution.

Probiotics are being promoted as an autism cure. The FDA says probiotics "have not been proven safe and effective for these advertised uses."

————

Here's how the FDA suggests you avoid fraudulent claims:

- Be suspicious of products that claim to treat a wide range of diseases.

- Personal testimonials are not a substitute for scientific evidence.

- Few diseases or conditions can be treated quickly, so be suspicious of any therapy claimed as a "quick fix."

- So-called miracle cures, which claim scientific breakthroughs and secret ingredients, are probably a hoax.

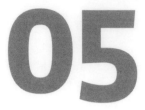

Are children being paralyzed by the common cold virus?

n August 2014, a child was taken to Children's Hospital Colorado in Aurora, Colorado, by frantic parents. The child had been fine one moment and paralyzed the next. Doctors couldn't figure out why a perfectly healthy child would suddenly be unable to stand up and walk. Before they could figure out what was going on, another child was brought into the hospital. And another.

Next came a baby who was floppy. Then a child whose breathing muscles were paralyzed and who had to be intubated and put on a ventilator. By September 17, eight more children at Children's Hospital Colorado were paralyzed or suffering weakness. By the end of October, there were twelve. Nearly all had suffered a minor cold in the days before paralysis.

Across the country, a hundred more families were living the same horror: previously active children were suddenly slurring their speech and struggling to walk and breathe. Doctors diagnosed them with a rare condition called acute flaccid myelitis, or AFM, a destructive disease of the spinal cord, specifically the part known as gray matter. AFM usually affects fewer than one in a million people in the United States each year. Cases are sporadic and spread out.

By December 2014, 120 children in thirty-four states had been diagnosed with AFM. The next year, twenty-two children were paralyzed in the same pattern—each suffered a mild cold before paralysis. In 2016, 153 children were confirmed to have AFM. The outbreak followed a biennial pattern. Every other year more than a hundred children became paralyzed after a cold infection in the late summer and fall. In 2018, 237 children were confirmed to have AFM. The 601 cases confirmed between 2014 and 2019 were mostly boys. The average age of the paralyzed children was 5 years. Pediatricians, neurologists, and disease detectives could not decipher the medical mystery.

AFM can be caused by viruses including poliovirus and West Nile virus as well as environmental toxins or the body's own immune system attacking nerve cells. The disease causes sudden onset weakness and paralysis, including drooping eyelids, weak reflexes, loss of muscle tone, slurred speech, and difficulty swallowing. In severe cases, the muscles of breathing are paralyzed and a person can suffocate to death.

There is no treatment for AFM, only supportive measures such as assisted breathing with ventilators and in a few cases, a special surgery to stabilize the hip joint and help regain some movement of the legs.

For terrified parents wondering if their children would ever walk again, there were few answers. The long-term prognosis for AFM is unknown.

At the same time that the unusual outbreak of AFM was spreading across the country, another epidemic was simmering. The United States was experiencing its largest ever outbreak of enterovirus D68, or EV-D68, a virus that causes coldlike symptoms. Between 1970 and 2005, twenty-six cases of EV-D68 were reported in the United States. In 2014, that number shot up to 1,153, including fourteen deaths. The virus went from a few states to appearing in forty-nine states and the District of Columbia.

Parents of the children paralyzed in the fall of 2014 said many had come down with a cold in the days before they were diagnosed with AFM. When investigators at the Centers for Disease Control and Prevention tested fluid from the children's nasal passages for EV-D68, they found the virus in almost half of children who had specimens collected within seven days' onset of fever or respiratory illness.

Astute doctors were connecting the dots. Two nationwide outbreaks were happening at the same time, and they wondered if AFM and EV-D68 were linked. Could a usually mild respiratory virus suddenly be causing nerve damage in children? Could the virus have changed to infect a different type of cell to cause an entirely different kind of disease?

Investigators at the CDC asked doctors across the country to send samples from the children's nasal passages as well as samples of cerebrospinal fluid, or CSF, the fluid surrounding the spinal cord. If EV-D68 was damaging the spinal cord, they expected to find the virus in the fluid drained during a spinal tap. But only one child had CSF that tested positive for EV-D68.

For some doctors, that didn't rule out the possibility that the virus was implicated in many more cases. EV-D68 contains RNA, DNA's more fragile cousin. RNA degrades quickly when sampled in a spinal tap. "Literally from the time it hits the tube to walking to the lab, the RNA could be all gone," said Dr. Benjamin Greenberg, a neurologist at UT Southwestern Medical Center in Dallas, who treated children with AFM in the 2014 outbreak.

The cluster of cases that began with twelve children at Children's Hospital Colorado in August 2014 and ended the year with 120 children diagnosed with AFM, wasn't the first clustering of AFM in the United States. At a meeting of the American Academy of Neurology in Philadelphia in April 2014, doctors from California reported seeing something similar years earlier.

Beginning in the fall of 2012, doctors at Lucile Packard Children's Hospital at Stanford University saw five children with AFM. Two of them had EV-D68 in their nasal passages.

Later that year, in August 2012, California doctors treated a 29-year-old man with AFM. They alerted the California Department of Public Health. Within the next two weeks, the health department received two more reports. By the summer of 2013, five children in California had presented with sudden onset paralysis. Three of the children had a respiratory illness in the days before they became paralyzed. Two children tested positive for EV-D68.

The numbers kept increasing. By May 2014, twenty-three people across California had been diagnosed with AFM. By the summer of 2015, the number was fifty-nine. Nine of the forty-one who were tested for EV-D68 in their nasal passages tested positive. None had the virus in the fluid surrounding their spinal cords.

ENTEROVIRUS OR SOMETHING ELSE?

Not everyone was convinced that EV-D68 was the culprit in the national out-break of paralysis. The CDC was casting its net wide and testing patients for many other viruses, including West Nile virus. Poliovirus was ruled out as a cause early on.

But some scientists were frustrated with this approach. They argued that with so many patients complaining of coldlike symptoms in the days before paralysis and many of them testing positive for the virus, the CDC should nar-row its focus and resources on investigating EV-D68 as the most likely culprit.

Others believed an entirely new pathogen, yet to be identified, was to blame. Some pointed the finger at the immune system, saying if it was fired up after infection, it could mistakenly unleash its anger on nerve cells, which is exactly what happens with another paralytic illness called Guillain-Barré syndrome. People usually become paralyzed with Guillain-Barré syndrome in the days after a mild stomach infection with a bacteria transmitted through food.

But EV-D68 remained the most popular theory behind the nationwide out-break of AFM, and scientists began taking a closer look at the virus.

Enteroviruses get their name from the ancient Greek word *enteron,* meaning "intestine," since they are transmitted through the gut, although they are also shed in respiratory secretions. The viruses are part of a virus family known as picornaviridae, *pico* meaning "small" and *rna* for the single strand of genetic material they carry. You might have heard of the most famous enterovirus, poliovirus, which causes paralysis and even death, as well as rhinovirus, the most common cause of the cold.

Enteroviruses are split into two groups, polioviruses and nonpoliovirus-es. Among the nonpolioviruses are rhinoviruses, which cause the common cold year-round, as well as other enteroviruses that cause the common "sum-mer cold," especially in children, since they haven't had the chance to build up immunity.

EV-D68 was first discovered in California in 1962 in specimens taken from four children with pneumonia and bronchiolitis. While EV-D68 was found to cause mild symptoms such as fever, cough, a runny nose, and in a few cases, chest infections, other enteroviruses are known to cause more severe illnesses, including swelling of the lining of the brain, infection of the heart and hand, and foot and mouth disease. Some of the nonpolio enteroviruses cause paralysis. EV-A71 and EV-D70 cause an acute flaccid paralysis that does long-term damage and which some people don't fully recover from.

Scientists wondered if the strain of EV-D68 circulating in the United States in 2014 had changed in some way from the strain that usually caused a mild cold. Could the virus have shifted its appetite and become more dangerous? Different viruses enter and infect different cells. HIV loves cells of the immune system, in particular, T cells. Dengue viruses like white blood cells called dendritic cells and monocytes. Human T cell leukemia viruses infect blood cells, and flu has a predilection for the cells that line the respiratory tract.

EV-D68 was known to have that same preference for cells of the upper respiratory tract, but in 2018 scientists at the National Institutes of Health discovered that the strain of EV-D68 circulating throughout the United States in 2014 was indeed different from the strain isolated in a California lab in 1962. The virus had "undergone significant evolutionary shifts" since then, the scientists wrote. This new strain of EV-D68 had acquired the ability to enter nerve cells, replicate inside, and potentially kill them.

Like humans, viruses have family trees with different branches. In the 1990s, the EV-D68 family tree split into two groups, or what virologists call clades. These two groups were labeled A and C. In the early 2000s, clade C split into a third group called clade B. In 2010, a new clade, B1, separated from group B. It was this group of EV-D68 virus, clade B1, that was the main culprit in the 2014 outbreak.

To see if the new strain of EV-D68, group B1, could infect nerve cells, scientists at the National Institutes of Health and Vanderbilt University tried adding it to cells taken from a cancer of nerve tissue, called neuroblastoma. When they added the 1962 strain of EV-D68, there was no infection of the nerve cells. But when they added the newer strain of EV-D68, the strain that caused the 2014 outbreak, the virus entered the cells and replicated inside them.

There were genetic changes in the virus, too. A group of scientists at the University of California, San Diego, discovered that the RNA of the outbreak strain of EV-D68 was different from older strains of the virus. In fact, the newer strain of EV-D68 had twenty-one changes and a genetic code more in line with enteroviruses such as EV-D70 and EV-A71, which can cause paralysis. "Based on these results, we hypothesize that unique B1 substitutions may be responsible for the apparent increased incidence of neuropathology associated with the 2014 outbreak," they said.

Mice infected with the outbreak strain of EV-D68 became paralyzed, but not mice infected with the 1962 strain. Alison Hixon, a scientist at the University of Colorado, made this discovery in 2017, when she injected the different strains of EV-D68 into mouse brains. Using strains of the virus from people sickened in the 2014 outbreak, she proved that in mice, it was the new strain, clade B1, that had the ability to cause damage and even kill spinal cord nerve cells. Under a microscope, she saw that the outbreak strain caused a loss of motor neurons in the anterior horn of the spinal cord, which was exactly the part of the spinal cord damaged in children with AFM.

CAUSALITY

But were these experiments in petri dishes and mice enough to prove the virus was causing paralysis? Epidemiologists are very careful about uttering the words *cause* or *causation.* Instead, we use terms like *associated* or *linked* or *correlated,* because it can be tricky to say one thing causes another. You may have heard the phrase: association is not the same as causation. Or, correlation does not imply causation. Many studies can tell us two things are linked, but it's harder to say one causes the other. Just because two epidemics were occurring in the same place at the same time, doesn't mean one epidemic was causing the other.

In the nineteenth century, when miasma, evil spirits, and humors were believed to cause illness, a German doctor and microbiologist set out four criteria that could be used to say a pathogen was the cause of disease. Robert Koch's four criteria have come to be known as Koch's postulates.

Koch's postulates say that for a particular microbe to be determined as the cause of illness, the organism must be regularly associated with the disease; it must be isolated from the host with the disease and grown in culture; the disease must be reproduced when a healthy person is exposed to a pure culture of the organism; and the same organism must be reisolated from the person who was infected with that culture.

Koch's postulates placed the science of microbiology on solid ground. No more blaming the stars, evil spirits, or bad air. Koch laid out exactly how a pathogen could be proven as the causative agent of a disease. He used his postulates to show that tuberculosis in humans was caused by bacteria different from the bug that caused anthrax in cattle.

But his criteria weren't foolproof. What about pathogens that are difficult to grow in culture? What about those pathogens that are found in healthy people and don't cause illness in everyone? Koch himself identified microbes that were the likely cause of illness but did not meet his four criteria. There was *Vibrio cholerae*, which causes cholera but which can be isolated from healthy people as well as those who are sick, a phenomenon that invalidated the second postulate.

Then there was the question of viruses. Viruses don't cause illness in everyone infected, they can be difficult to isolate and grow in the lab, and some viruses lack good animal models for their study.

Viruses hadn't been discovered when Koch devised his four postulates, and these days virologists have a longer list of postulates based on Koch's writings but with a healthy dose of technology added. In 1996, two scientists came up with a seven-point "reconsideration of Koch's postulates." David Relman and David Fredricks included the requirement that the DNA or RNA of the pathogen should be present in most cases of the disease.

In the case of EV-D68, it hasn't been found in every child suffering with AFM, and it likely would be found in healthy people, if we went looking for it. Scientists expected to find the virus floating in the cerebrospinal fluid of children with damaged spinal cords but found it in only a few cases. Is that enough to say the virus is not the cause of the outbreak?

Not according to doctors at the University of Colorado. They applied a different set of criteria, known as the Bradford Hill criteria. In a paper published in the *Lancet* in August 2018, the doctors said there was a causal relationship between EV-D68 and AFM.

In 1965 Sir Austin Bradford Hill, a British epidemiologist and one-half of the duo who established that smoking causes cancer, asked this question: "In what circumstances can one pass from observed association to a verdict of causation?"

Bradford Hill proposed nine "aspects of association" for evaluating traditional epidemiologic data. Unlike Koch's postulates, all nine of the Bradford Hill criteria do not have to be met for a verdict of causation to be made. In the 2018 paper in the *Lancet,* doctors at the University of Colorado went through each of the nine Bradford Hill criteria in the context of EV-D68 and AFM and said seven of the nine criteria were met.

First, there was a temporal association. Many children with AFM had a fever or respiratory illness in the days before they became paralyzed. Some tested positive for the infection in the early days of paralysis.

Second, there was plausibility. In a 5-year-old boy who died in 2011 from swelling of the brain and spinal cord, an autopsy showed EV-D68 in the fluid surrounding the spinal cord.

Third, there was consistency. Infection with EV-D68 has been linked to AFM, mostly in children, in fourteen countries around the world, including Argentina, Australia, Italy, France, Norway, Canada, and elsewhere.

Fourth, there was coherence. Studies had shown a newer strain of the virus can infect nerve cells. And fifth, experiments showed newer strains caused paralysis in mice by damaging motor neurons in the spinal cord.

Sixth, there was strength of association, since EV-D68 was the virus most commonly isolated from people suffering with AFM in 2014 and 2016. Finally, the clinical presentation of AFM associated with EV-D68, the children's MRIs, and other diagnostic findings were similar to that seen in the paralysis caused by other enteroviruses and polioviruses.

There was no biological gradient, the doctors wrote, since there was no dose-response relationship and some children with severe paralysis had very low levels of EV-D68 in respiratory samples. There was also no specificity. Various enteroviruses such as EV-D70 and EV-A71 are known to cause paralysis, and EV-D68 is thought to mostly cause a respiratory illness, not AFM.

ANOTHER OUTBREAK OF PARALYSIS

When an outbreak of paralysis among children emerged in the fall of 2018, parents, doctors, and scientists voiced their fears and frustrations. It had been six years since one of the first epidemics of AFM had occurred in the United

States and four years since doctors had rung the alarm bell. Why hadn't more been done to pinpoint the cause of the outbreak? Why wasn't there a vaccine for the new strain of EV-D68?

Doctors accused the CDC of being slow to gather data and slow to give them guidance on how to manage AFM in emergency rooms and on pediatric wards. Scientists, even those advising the CDC, said the agency was casting its net too wide and not focusing on the most likely culprit: EV-D68.

By January 2020, 603 children were confirmed to have AFM, and some children were said to have died months after developing the disease, although the number was not released. Some scientists demanded that AFM be added to the list of diseases that have to be reported to the CDC. But surveillance for that kind of paralysis ended in the United States with the regional eradication of polio in the mid-twentieth century. Perhaps it was time to resurrect that surveillance system, some scientists said, and to begin active surveillance of EV-D68.

The number of children diagnosed with AFM in the United States begins to creep upward in the late summer with a spike in the fall. It's a pattern that repeats every other year.

For parents, the advice for combating the mysterious and frightening disease remains simple—almost frustratingly so. To ward off a new disease that starts with a fever and runny nose but can turn into paralysis: wash your children's hands with soap and water.

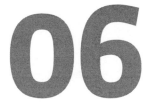

Do we inherit trauma from our parents?

In the fall of 2015, Rachel Yehuda and her team at the Icahn School of Medicine at Mount Sinai in New York published results of a study looking at the genes of thirty-two Jewish women and men. All were Holocaust survivors who either had been interned in Nazi concentration camps, forced into hiding during World War II, or seen or experienced torture. The team also studied the genes of twenty-two children who were born to Holocaust survivors after the war.

Previous studies had found that children of Holocaust survivors have a higher risk of developing post-traumatic stress disorder, depression, and anxiety, especially if the parents themselves have PTSD. In a 2015 paper in the journal *Biological Psychiatry*, Yehuda wrote that she had found a genetic explanation for this apparent inheritance of trauma.

Her team was looking to see if changes to the offspring's DNA were due to trauma the offspring had suffered directly. But they couldn't find that link. They concluded that changes to the offspring's DNA were due to the suffering their parents endured during the Holocaust.

What Yehuda described is known as epigenetic inheritance. It's the idea that traumatic experiences affect DNA in ways that are passed on to children and grandchildren, kind of like molecular scars.

If DNA contains instructions for making eyes brown and hair curly, epigenetics refers to ways in which those genes are turned on and off. Genes are the blueprint for creating proteins. Epigenetics is the study of how genes are read.

An epigenetic change is one that sits on the DNA, not in it, affecting the way genes function without changing the genes themselves. The idea has taken off, and New Age guru Deepak Chopra is among those who support the finding.

At least that's the original definition of *epigenetics*. Nowadays, the term is also used to describe gene modifications that are passed on from parents to children. Some scientists say we transmit more than our genes. We also pass on molecular switches and information about how those genes should be expressed.

One of the most studied epigenetic modifications is DNA methylation. It's where small molecules are added to genes, changing the activity of DNA. In a study published in the *American Journal of Psychiatry* in 2014, Yehuda found that male Holocaust survivors who suffered PTSD had children with higher methylation of a gene involved in the stress response.

But these changes are exceedingly difficult to interpret. Yehuda's team found that if both of the child's parents were Holocaust survivors with PTSD, the child was more likely to have lower methylation of that gene. It's unknown if that epigenetic change was shared directly from a sperm or egg, or if it took place in the uterus as the baby developed, or in early childhood.

The problems with Yehuda's 2015 study—which is still generating headlines stating that trauma is inherited, despite her team's best efforts to clarify the science—begin with the small study size. Only thirty-two survivors and twenty-two of their offspring were studied. That's a very small group on which to base this theory and a major study flaw that many media outlets overlooked. Yehuda's team were transparent about the limitations of studying such a small group of people, and Yehuda described her studies as the beginning of a long line of experiments needed to understand this phenomenon.

While the team studied the children of women who lived through the Holocaust, they would have to study the great-grandchildren of survivors to prove actual epigenetic inheritance from mother to offspring. Why must four generations be studied? Baby girls are born with their lifetime supply of eggs. The egg that made you was present inside your mother when she was a fetus inside your grandmother. Because a pregnant woman already possesses the DNA of her grandchildren and these genes can be affected by things during her pregnancy, the DNA of the great-grandchildren has to be studied to show that epigenetic changes were passed on across generations.

The study also focused on a very small number of genes. And it didn't account for the influence of social factors. Children born to Holocaust survivors may grow up listening to accounts of the war's horrors. Josie Glausiusz, a participant in Yehuda's 2014 study, raised this point in an essay in the Israeli newspaper *Haaretz*. Glausiusz's father survived the Bergen-Belsen concentration camp. She wrote, "I was troubled by a question: How does one separate the impact of horrific stories heard in childhood from the influence of epigenetics?" She's not the only one to raise this question. Yehuda has asked it herself.

Other researchers have cast doubt on the study's conclusions based on the small changes in DNA methylation that were seen. Then there's the issue of reverse causation: If DNA methylation is significant, is that change caused by trauma or does the methylation itself increase the risk of PTSD?

The week after the study was published, the blog of the Center for Epigenomics at the Albert Einstein College of Medicine in New York called it the "over-interpreted epigenetics study of the week."

Which was true. Reporters ran with the results from a small study, overlooking the caution offered by the researchers.

John Greally, professor of genetics at the college, wrote: "The story being told by the Holocaust study is indeed fascinating as a scientific possibility, and will no doubt prompt others to pursue similar studies. Unfortunately, the story is typical of many in the field of epigenetics, with conclusions drawn based on uninterpretable studies."

Those who survived the horrors of the Holocaust and other tragedies find themselves asking if they will pass that trauma on to their children. The headlines say yes but based on a close look at the research, the answer so far is no.

07

Are genetically modified foods safe?

G enetically modified foods are not new. The term might conjure up images of Dolly the sheep, but we've been eating genetically modified food for millennia, ever since our ancestors bred this crop with that one to create genetically superior hybrids. According to some crop scientists: "Genetically modified food would include almost all the food we eat."

Sweet potatoes might not exist if it weren't for farmers breeding the roots of various potatoes thousands of years ago to make an entirely new and delicious kind. One scientific paper published by the National Academy of Sciences refers to sweet potatoes as "a naturally transgenic food crop."

How does it work? Let's clear up the terminology first. We use *genetically modified organism,* or GMO, and *genetically engineered* interchangeably, but they mean different things. Genetic modification refers to a range of methods such as hybridization and induced mutation, which are used to change the genome of an organism.

Genetic engineering is one kind of genetic modification. It uses biotechnology to directly manipulate an organism's genes. An example is corn that is engineered to be resistant to insects that would damage the crop.

Scientists take pieces of DNA from one organism, say, genes from Granny Smith and Golden Delicious apples. Then they change them, in our example by suppressing the enzyme responsible for turning apples brown. Then they put the genes into the leaf of the apples to make a new variety, Arctic apples, which don't turn brown.

The reinsertion part can be done using a gene gun that shoots pellets coated with DNA into the plant. Also known as microprojectile bombardment, the gene gun method uses pressurized gas and a vacuum chamber to force gene-coated metal particles into a cell's nucleus. Another way to modify genes is to use safe bacteria to deliver new or modified genetic material.

Genetic engineering doesn't necessarily involve taking genes from one species and putting them into a second species to create a transgenic organism. Sometimes genes are moved around within the same organism or a gene is moved from a closely related organism to make a cisgenic organism, as in the case of the Arctic apple. A third type of organism known as subgenic is made when genes are edited and either repressed, silenced, deleted, or inserted.

Before the discovery of sophisticated genetic engineering methods, scientists resorted to chemicals and radiation to make genetic changes in crops. It was messy and unreliable. More precise means to modify the genomes of foods have been around since the eighties, which might be why fear and suspicion cloak the world of GMOs. These technologies are relatively new.

In the 1980s, psychologist Robert Sternberg said humans consider the familiar to be natural and the unfamiliar to be unnatural. And maybe this question is at the heart of the issue: What is natural and what is unnatural?

I've been fascinated by this debate since the high school chemistry class where I learned the sweet scent of a strawberry (itself a hybrid species) comes from the chemical ethyl butanoate. How natural does that sound? And yet it is.

Some people are prone to calling GMOs frankenfoods, and more than a third of Americans believe genetically modified foods are "worse for one's health," according to a study by the Pew Research Center. That's perhaps without realizing that a punnet of garden strawberries from the farmer's market is a result of crossing a Chilean plant with a North American one in the eighteenth century—a type of genetic modification.

Eating genetically modified foods such as strawberries, corn, and sweet potatoes isn't bad for our health (unless we eat too many). Worries about poisoning our bodies, increasing allergies, or lowering the nutrition of foods have been studied through thousands of experiments, not to mention our daily consumption of modified foods over centuries.

Since GMOs landed on our shelves in the mid-nineties, scientists have searched for any harmful effects of eating them. None have been found so far. The World Health Organization says genetically modified foods have not been shown to cause harm. The National Academy of Sciences, the American Medical Association, and many other institutions take the same stance. There is no evidence that eating genetically modified food hurts adults or children.

In fact, when the genes of a plant are tinkered with to make it more resistant to insects, the yield of the crop increases, and fewer chemicals are sprayed. Genetically engineering corn to make it resistant to a common fungus boosts the yield of the crop, prevents the need for antifungal chemicals, and protects us and the plant from being exposed to the mold. The pesticide issue is a significant one for agricultural workers: every year 10,000 to 20,000 agricultural workers in the United States are diagnosed with pesticide poisoning.

One study making the rounds on anti-GMO websites claims that GMO corn causes cancer in rats. But the study was retracted a year after it was published when scientists pointed out mistakes and design flaws.

Besides safety checks, genetically modified foods are tested and compared to nongenetically modified foods for their vitamin and mineral contents. The nutritional value of genetically modified foods has not been found to be lower overall.

Some genetically modified foods are designed to fight famine and malnutrition or provide healthier alternatives. You may have seen canola oil labeled as low linoleic acid, which is designed to reduce its content of trans fats.

Then there's the yellow rice crop known as Golden Rice. Golden Rice is engineered to contain beta-carotene, a source of vitamin A in humans. Children in many parts of the world are weaned on regular rice and become deficient in vitamin A, which causes blindness and death from infections. One bowl of

Golden Rice provides a child with more than half their daily requirement of vitamin A. After years of arguing over its safety, Golden Rice was approved by the Food and Drug Administration in 2018.

Some controversies about GMOs remain unresolved. Take the case of genetically modified seeds for corn, alfalfa, cotton, and other crops that are made resistant to Roundup, the most commonly used herbicide in the world. These crops are known as Roundup Ready, and there are concerns that their use has allowed farmers to spray more Roundup on their crops knowing that the crops will be safe and weeds will be wiped out.

But weeds are wily. The active ingredient in Roundup, glyphosate, acts as a selective pressure on the weeds, meaning the weeds evolve and become resistant to the chemical meant to destroy them. Selective pressures drive natural selection. It's how people who lived in sunnier climes evolved to have darker skin, since melanin protects against damage from the sun's rays. The glyphosate-resistant weeds are an example of Darwinian evolution—on speed.

The GMO debate has become embroiled with the herbicide debate because the use of Roundup Ready crops has helped create so-called superweeds. Roundup, originally made by Monsanto in the 1970s and now sold by other manufacturers, is used by farmers and gardeners the world over. The scientific jury is still out on its safety, but in 2018, San Francisco jurors awarded a school groundsman $289 million when they ruled Roundup caused Dewayne Johnson's cancer.

While some were happy to see Monsanto punished, many scientists said the link between the chemical and the cancer is not proven. The World Health Organization says glyphosate is "probably carcinogenic in humans." Many studies have not found that to be true. Besides Johnson, 800 people are suing Monsanto claiming their cancers were caused by Roundup.

In lab rats, the active ingredient in Roundup, glyphosate, was linked to a higher risk of fatty liver disease, according to scientists in the United Kingdom. Although the impact of glyphosate in humans is not well understood, we do know it's turning up more frequently in our bodies.

The percentage of southern Californians testing positive for glyphosate went up 500 percent between 1993 to 2016, according to a study published in 2017. At the same time, levels of glyphosate went up 1,208 percent. These levels are 100 times higher than the levels found in the lab rats who developed liver disease.

Back to the GMO debate. The gene for glyphosate resistance hasn't been passed from the genetically engineered seeds to the weeds. The weeds are doing what they need to do in order to survive: developing resistance to glyphosate. But there is another concern about Roundup Ready seeds. Nicknamed "terminator seeds," these seeds produce sterile crops, which means farmers have to keep buying new seeds from Monsanto. This feeds into the idea of GMOs being the frankenbaby of evil megacorporations.

Although genes from the terminator seeds are not being spread to weeds, we know that many plants do like to share bits of DNA—they do it by spreading pollen. (Pollen is a bit like plant sperm.) There is fear that GMOs will spread their genes to wild plants to create new hybrids.

Here's why that doesn't concern many geneticists. In the case of superweeds resistant to glyphosate, the weeds are evolving to survive. But in the case of our genetically engineered Golden Rice and Arctic apples, they provide us with better nutrition and prettier apples without enhancing the organism's survival in the wild.

For genes to not only spread but to continue to be inherited through a plant's lineage, they have to offer advantage, otherwise they will be weeded out in favor of genes that boost a plant's chances of survival.

Genes from an Arctic apple, if they spread, are unlikely to boost an apple's resilience. And since genes that aid survival are the ones that are passed down, it's unlikely the gene for beta-carotene or apples that won't turn brown will continue to be passed along.

These GMOs can solve child blindness and food waste. Should they be thrown out because we fear the unknown? The case for the safety of GMOs might have to be made on a case by case basis: perhaps it's a yes to rice that can end child blindness, no to terminator seeds that create superweeds.

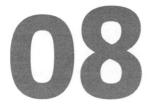

How long can you eat leftovers?

n July 2018, a few hundred residents of Powell, Ohio, began to feel sick. First there was stomach cramping, then there was diarrhea. Clayton Jones said he had eaten a burrito bowl from fast-food chain Chipotle on July 27 and fallen sick the next day. Filip Szyller bought three tacos at the same Chipotle store on July 29 and became sick on July 30. By August 6, 703 people said they were ill after eating at the same restaurant. The bacteria *Clostridium perfringens* was found in the stool samples of those who were tested. The bug grows in food that is kept warm for a long time before being served and is known to pop up in gravies, beef, and poultry when they are stored at the wrong temperature.

Every year, 48 million Americans—that's one in six people—suffers food poisoning. More than 128,000 are hospitalized as a result and 3,000 die. *C. perfringens* is responsible for almost a million cases of foodborne illness each year, making it one of the most common types of foodborne illness.

Foodborne outbreaks can be linked to farming practices and bad hygiene and food preparation in restaurants. Taco Bell, Wendy's, McDonald's, and Kentucky

Fried Chicken have all been at the center of food poisoning outbreaks. But it's not just fast food chains that are at risk of sickening patrons. A Michelin-starred restaurant in Valencia, Spain, closed after a food poisoning outbreak in 2019 that killed one woman and caused illness in twenty-nine diners.

Avoiding food poisoning at home requires translating ambiguous labels and distinguishing "best-before" dates from "best-by" dates. To reduce waste and avoid getting sick from what remains of dinner, follow this advice on how long to keep leftovers.

Baked ham, turkey, duck, and goose can be kept for three to four days in the fridge or two to three months in the freezer, but refrigerate or freeze leftovers within two hours of serving. Roast chicken keeps three to four days in the fridge or four months in the freezer. Remove stuffing from the bird before placing it in an airtight container in the fridge.

Sides such as mashed potatoes, yams, and green bean casserole last three to five days in the fridge and up to a year in the freezer. Gravy keeps for one to two days in the fridge and two to three months in the freezer. Don't drink eggnog more than a day after it was prepared, although it can be frozen for up to six months.

Pooling data from the US Department of Agriculture, the Food and Drug Administration, and the Centers for Disease Control and Prevention, the website StillTasty.com offers a searchable "Keep it or Toss it?" index to help you figure out which leftovers are safe to eat.

UNDERSTANDING EXPIRATION DATES

Only the expiration dates on baby food and infant formula are regulated by the government. If you see an "expires on" date on these items, follow the advice closely. But "best-by" and "best-before" dates tell you more about a food's optimal tastiness than they do its safety.

For example, take the best-by date on a jar of mustard or peanut butter. Even if it reads "best by Aug. 27," it's probably safe to eat in December as long as you have stored it unopened and at the correct temperature, though the quality may be reduced. That's because manufacturers voluntarily put dates on foods to indicate when they will taste best.

How can you tell if it's safe to eat? Use your nose. The highly scientific method of sniffing food is a decent way to detect if it is spoiled.

While best-by and best-before dates are found on shelf items such as mayonnaise, peanut butter, and mustard, perishable items such as meat and dairy usually have a sell-by date. The date is intended to offer guidance to stores as opposed to consumers.

That means you can still consume milk a week after the sell-by date, but only if it has been refrigerated the entire time. The same goes for ground meat, which can be eaten up to two days after the sell-by date, but again only if it has been continuously stored at the right temperature.

FOOD POISONING

Different bugs cause different symptoms and take varying amounts of time to make you sick. Salmonella and norovirus are the most common causes of food poisoning in the United States, according to the CDC. About six in ten outbreaks of food poisoning occur at restaurants, and about one in ten originates in the home.

Here's a guide to some of the most common causes of food poisoning:

Staphylococcus aureus is a bacteria found in meat that hasn't been kept at the right temperature, as well as egg and potato salads and cream pastries. It causes sudden vomiting and stomach cramps, and some people also suffer fever and diarrhea. Symptoms begin within six hours after exposure.

Vibrio parahaemolyticus is a bacteria found in raw or undercooked seafood, especially shellfish. It causes stomach cramps, vomiting, fever, and watery diarrhea four to ninety-six hours after exposure.

Salmonella is found in eggs, poultry, unpasteurized milk, juice, and cheese. It causes fever, stomach cramps, diarrhea, and vomiting twelve to seventy-two hours after exposure.

Clostridium perfringens is a bacteria that causes severe stomach cramps and watery diarrhea. It is found in meat and gravy and causes symptoms eight to sixteen hours after the contaminated food is eaten.

Listeria is a bacteria found in unpasteurized dairy products and some deli meats. It causes fever, diarrhea, and muscle aches. In pregnant women, even those with mild symptoms, listeria can cause miscarriage or stillbirth. In the elderly or people with a weakened immune system, the bacteria can infect the bloodstream and lining of the brain.

Norovirus is very contagious and spreads through person-to-person contact and contaminated food when an infected person doesn't wash his or her hands. Shellfish in water containing the virus can also cause illness, as well as raw and undercooked foods. Symptoms begin twelve to forty-eight hours after exposure and include diarrhea, vomiting, fever, and headache. Adults are more likely to suffer diarrhea, and children are more likely to suffer vomiting.

Clostridium botulinum is an extremely dangerous bacteria that produces a potent nerve toxin that can paralyze muscles and cause death. The toxin is found in improperly canned foods, so if you can foods at home, follow instructions carefully. Botulism can also result if you bake a potato in foil and then store it in the foil.

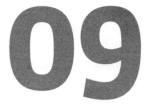

Is MSG addictive?

I grew up with a mysterious white substance sprinkled and stirred into our home-cooked Indian food. Labeled Aji No Moto, it sat in a glass jar on a shelf packed full of Indian and Burmese spices. It wasn't until I was an adult that I realized Aji No Moto was another name for MSG, or monosodium gluta-mate, the dreaded additive said to be addictive and unhealthy. I was horrified. Racing hearts, anxiety, sluggishness, and brain fog were supposed side effects of eating the stuff and I had grown up eating it. MSG was blamed for a variety of ailments and became synonymous with take-out Chinese food, which we were told was full of the white crystals.

It was all lies. The health claims made about MSG were debunked starting in the 1960s, but the stereotypes of Chinese food as addictive and unhealthy persisted, and people still avoid MSG for fear of harmful health effects.

The MSG story starts in 1907, when Kikunae Ikeda, a Japanese chemist, was trying to find the element that gave foods like seaweed and asparagus their distinct flavor. Ikeda discovered that an amino acid called glutamate was responsible for the yumminess and discovered a way to make it by extracting the amino acid from seaweed. He added the glutamate to salt, found a way to stabilize the formula and patented his discovery in 1909. MSG was born.

A few decades later, so was "Chinese Restaurant Syndrome." Also known as CRS, the syndrome was sometimes referred to as post-sinocibal syndrome in the medical literature where it first appeared in 1968. That year Dr. Robert Ho Man Kwok, a Chinese doctor living in the United States, wrote a letter to the editors of the *New England Journal of Medicine* describing the illness he felt after eating Chinese food in American restaurants. Kwok said he felt a "numbness at the back of the neck, gradually radiating to both arms and the back, general weakness and palpitation." These symptoms started twenty minutes or so after he ate food from American Chinese restaurants, so the doctor proposed that his symptoms were caused by food that was prepared with Chinese cooking wine, too much salt, or MSG.

Many more people wrote to the medical journal to back up Kwok's claims. But they were missing a crucial point. By pointing the finger at Chinese food, they were ignoring that MSG was added to all kinds of cuisines by people all around the world. In fact, MSG wasn't a new ingredient that had suddenly appeared in North America in the 1960s. It had been around in the United States and Canada since the end of World War II. My family, who emigrated to England from India, had been using it since the 1970s.

Still, the fact that "Chinese Restaurant Syndrome" was appearing in prestigious medical journals, and that it had a fancy medical name, fueled a fear of ethnic food in the West. It didn't matter that researchers were publishing papers showing the additive didn't cause palpitations or pain that radiated down the arms and neck.

Food historians who study MSG and Chinese Restaurant Syndrome say this could be due to three things: the availability heuristic, the nocebo effect, and racism. Or all three.

The availability heuristic happens when we make judgments about something using information that's easiest to come across, whether that's rumors or hearsay, and when we don't consider other explanations. You could argue it was easy to jump to the conclusion that MSG was bad for you because everyone was saying so, and even those scientists publishing papers saying it wasn't bad were still studying it in the first place, so something must have been wrong. It didn't help that Chinese restaurants felt compelled to write "No MSG used here" on window signs and in menus.

The nocebo effect is the opposite of the more famous placebo effect, which you have probably heard about. The placebo effect happens when you take something that doesn't have any medical effects but makes you feel better because you believe it's good for you, and the nocebo effect is the opposite. A nocebo is something that also doesn't give any health effects but makes you feel worse when you take it because of your belief that it's bad for you.

Then there's racism, which could explain MSG's bad rap. Chinese cooks were using much more MSG than white people used, some said. This fed into racist stereotypes of Chinese immigrants as strange, unhygienic, and unhealthy.

Canadian historian of food and colonialism, Ian Mosby, who has written about MSG and Chinese Restaurant Syndrome, has also documented other food scares linked to Chinese food in the West. This includes scares about meat served in Chinatown in Vancouver even when there were no proven cases of ill people eating in those restaurants. About CRS, Mosby writes that it was a "unique medical condition . . . a disease whose spread owed as much to persisting prejudices about Chinese culinary practices and culture as it did to fears of the effects of MSG and other food additives."

The claims that Chinese cooks were using "lavish" amounts of MSG compared to white people were unfounded, Mosby writes. Nobody was conducting studies comparing how many grams of MSG Chinese cooks used when preparing food in restaurants.

It didn't matter. The belief that eating in Chinese restaurants could make you sick persisted long enough to put many people off eating MSG, despite studies that showed it was not toxic to humans. Perhaps that science could be doubted, since some of the studies claiming MSG is safe were done by companies that make MSG. That's a red flag for any study, and the findings should be taken with a pinch of salt.

In rats, chronic exposure to MSG is linked to kidney damage, and mice fed MSG developed kidney stones. But the additive remains on the "generally recognized as safe" food list, compiled by the Food and Drug Administration. The agency has extensively reviewed MSG, perhaps more so than other additives, because of the popularity of the concern over its safety and media coverage of those health concerns.

"Over the years, FDA has received reports of symptoms such as headache and nausea after eating foods containing MSG. However, we were never able to confirm that the MSG caused the reported effects," the agency writes on its website. In the 1990s it asked the Federation of American Societies for Experimental Biology, an independent group of scientists, to review the evidence. The scientists said it was safe to eat MSG.

It can be hard to dislodge bad science from the brain. Racist connotations of MSG persist, and it's not uncommon to hear someone say they avoid MSG because of its negative health effects. But those claims originated from awful stereotypes of Chinese cooks and say a lot more about the pervasiveness of racism than the health effects of a lab-made flavor enhancer.

10

Is drinking diet soda linked to Alzheimer's disease and stroke?

When a study said diet sodas were linked to brain diseases, it seemed you were damned if you drank sugary drinks and damned if you switched over to artificially sweetened ones. A 2017 study that followed thousands of people over a decade and tracked their beverage intake and brain health found people who drank diet soda every day were more likely to suffer dementia, particularly Alzheimer's disease, and stroke.

Alzheimer's disease is a type of dementia caused by bundles of sticky proteins and tangles of a toxic protein called tau. The proteins clump together in the brain and cause brain cells to die. Early symptoms of Alzheimer's include memory loss and problems remembering recently learned information. The disease progresses slowly to confusion, changes in behavior, and problems walking and swallowing, which can cause death when food is inhaled instead of swallowed properly and pneumonia ensues.

Stroke, where the blood supply to the brain is lost and the tissue starved of oxygen, was more likely in people who drank artificially sweetened drinks, the researchers said. In particular, ischemic stroke, the most common kind, which happens when arteries that feed the brain are blocked, was more common in diet soda drinkers.

Overall, the risk of stroke or dementia was nearly three times higher for people who drank one artificially sweetened soda a day, compared to those who drank less than one diet soda a week.

The study did not prove that artificial sweeteners cause stroke, Alzheimer's disease, or any type of dementia. Some of the headlines said otherwise. But this kind of study design cannot prove causation. To be fair, the authors were careful to say that the study was not "able to prove cause and effect and only shows a trend among one group of people." Many news articles didn't reflect this.

The researchers studied nearly 3,000 men and women ages 45 and older for stroke and about 1,500 people over age 60 for dementia. They tracked how much and what kinds of soda the subjects were drinking and monitored their health for a decade.

But what does diet soda have to do with your brain? We don't really know, not in humans anyway. In rats, the artificial sweetener aspartame inhibits an enzyme called creatine kinase. Scientists have found that aspartame interferes with the brain's energy production and the amount of electrolytes in the bloodstream. Soda-drinking rats had higher levels of sodium and calcium in the blood and lower levels of copper, iron, zinc, and potassium. But looking at those experiments it was hard to separate what was directly linked to aspartame and what might have been happening because of other chemicals in the sodas the rats were drinking.

Aspartame was approved by the Food and Drug Administration for use in food in 1981 and as a sweetener in 1996. It's a popular additive but remains controversial.

One clue to aspartame's effects on the brain comes from one of its three main components, phenylalanine, which regulates neurotransmitters. Another component, aspartic acid, is an excitatory neurotransmitter. The third component is methanol, which can be broken down by the body into some toxic chemicals.

But studies in humans have produced mixed results. When ninety university students answered questions about memory, students who used aspartame regularly said they had memory lapses. But studies like this one are small and rely on people's perceptions of their ability to remember information.

The study of diet soda drinkers published in the journal *Stroke* had some major caveats. First, the study didn't look at people's consumption of artificial sweeteners in things other than soft drinks. People who were classed as nondrinkers of diet soda could have been adding artificial sweeteners such as Sweet'N Low to yogurt, desserts, or tea and coffee.

Speaking of Sweet'N Low, it contains saccharin, one of the sweeteners approved by the FDA at the time of this decade-long study. Aspartame and acesulfame-K were also FDA-approved sweeteners at that time. But sucralose was approved in 1999, neotame in 2000, and stevia in 2008, after the study was completed. The scientists note this limitation, saying that "these synthetic substances are much more potent than sucrose, with only trace amounts needed to generate the sensation of sweetness." That means people using newer sweeteners might be exposed to much smaller amounts of the chemicals compared to those included in the study who used older, less potent artificial sweeteners.

It's important to bear in mind that drinkers of sugary sodas may have died from other causes such as heart disease and complications of diabetes, and that's why they don't show up in the results section as victims of stroke and dementia. This phenomenon is known as survival bias. Not mentioning it can be misleading.

And it could be the case that people who drink diet sodas every day are avoiding sugar because they already have other illnesses, such as diabetes or high blood pressure. Those diseases themselves are risk factors for stroke. That phenomenon as known as reverse causation.

In a different study by the same researchers involving around 4,000 people, those who drank sugary drinks such as sodas and fruit juice were found to have a smaller brain volume, as well as smaller hippocampi, the two horseshoe-shaped parts of the brain that are crucial to memory. In that study, which was published in the *Journal of the Alzheimer's Association*, people who drank sugary drinks were more likely to have memory problems. One or two sugar-filled beverages a day was linked with 1.6 years of brain aging. Drinking more than that was linked with two years of brain aging. When the researchers focused on memory specifically, drinking one or two sugary drinks a day was linked to nearly six years of brain aging, they said, and eleven years of brain aging for people who drank more than two sugary drinks a day.

The artificial sweetener study published in the journal *Stroke* emphasized the "relative risk" of stroke and dementia in people who drink diet sodas every day. One problem with reporting results using the relative risk is that it can make the likelihood of something happening seem bigger than it truly is. Relative risk tells you how more or less likely a disease occurs in one group compared with another. Relative risk does not tell you the actual likelihood that something will happen to you.

A better measurement is "absolute risk," which tells you your actual risk of developing a disease. Where the relative risk says the risk of dementia and stroke is three times higher in one group, the absolute risk says the actual likelihood of developing stroke and dementia in your lifetime is quite low. For example, in the group of people the researchers were monitoring for a decade, 3 percent suffered a stroke and 5 percent developed dementia.

Previous studies have found that artificial sweeteners interfere with good bacteria in the gut and are linked to weight gain and diseases of the veins and arteries.

"To our knowledge, our study is the first to report an association between daily intake of artificially sweetened soft drink and increased risk of both all-cause dementia and dementia because of Alzheimer's disease," the researchers said.

This doesn't mean that sugary sodas are a healthier option. Almost a third of Americans drink one or more sugary sodas or sweetened drinks a day, according to a 2016 report by the Centers for Disease Control and Prevention. Diets high in sugar are linked to heart disease, obesity, and diabetes, among other conditions.

So it's easy to see why you would want to switch from a sugar-filled soda to a diet one. The dangers of too much sugar are pretty well understood, and switching from a can of Coke a day to Diet Coke reduces your calorie intake by around 4,000 calories a month.

While this study doesn't prove that sugary sodas cause stroke and dementia, the scientists did say their results call for more research on the health effects of artificial sweeteners. And the missing link about exactly how artificial sweeteners might be harming the brain needs to be filled in, too. In the meantime, you might want to give up drinking soda altogether.

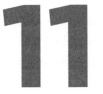

Do mammograms cause more problems than they detect?

Breast cancer is the most common cancer in women worldwide. It kills more than half a million women each year. So cancer screening sounds like a great idea—finding a cancer early before symptoms appear and before it spreads should increase the odds of survival and offer more treatment options—but it's not so straightforward.

The controversy begins with a Canadian study in the 1980s. Nearly 90,000 women aged 40 to 59 years were split into groups. Half received annual mammograms, half did not.

Mammograms, discovered in the early 1900s and first introduced in the 1970s, use low-energy x-rays to check for breast disease. The aim is to find small tumors before they become so big that they cause symptoms and spread to other parts of the body, allowing for treatment to start earlier and a person's life to be extended. Mammograms can't prove that a woman has breast cancer. They help doctors find lumps too small to be felt and decide whether further tests such as biopsies are needed.

In the Canadian study, mammograms were used to detect small tumors. But if the hope was that mammograms would find disease early and reduce cancer deaths, that wasn't happening. The Canadian study showed mammograms did not save lives.

A follow-up of the Canadian study published in 2014 looking at the same women for a further twenty-five years, found mammograms were not lowering the death rate from cancer. One study published in the *New England Journal of Medicine* in 2012 found that women who had mammograms were just as likely to die as women who didn't have mammograms.

Mammography misses about one in five cancers, according to the National Cancer Institute. For every 1,000 women who have a mammogram, 100 will have to go back for follow-up testing because of a suspicious finding. But of those 100, only five will have breast cancer.

This graph from a 2016 study in the *New England Journal of Medicine* shows the incidence of metastatic breast cancer (the stubborn bottom line) has remained stable even since mammograms were introduced for routine breast screening (see the figure). It means the number of women with cancer that spreads has not been reduced by mammograms.

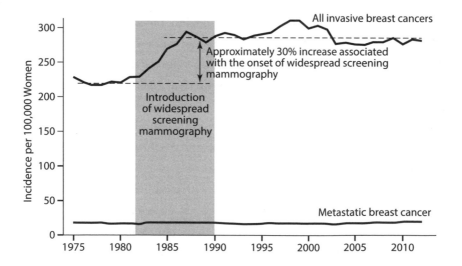

Incidences of invasive breast cancer and metastatic breast cancer in women aged 40 years and older from 1975 to 2012. Mammograms were rarely used before 1980 but widely used as a screening tool by 1990. *Data are from nine sites of the Surveillance, Epidemiology, and End Results study.*

In fact, screening with mammograms has been causing some women harm. In the same study, researchers found mammograms can lead to unnecessary overtreatment of nonharmful breast lumps. For every woman who may have had her life saved by a mammogram, four women were found to have tumors that may never have become serious.

One-fifth of invasive breast cancers detected by mammograms in this study were overdiagnosed. So for every 424 women screened in the trial, one woman was overdiagnosed with breast cancer and potentially received unnecessary treatment.

Overdiagnosis is the detection of cancers that are harmless and would not cause illness during a patient's life. Cancer screening raises tricky ethical and clinical questions about what to do when you see a mass that might be cancer . . . but might not be. Better to err on the side of caution and treat aggressively, you might think. But overdiagnosis leads to overtreatment. Women are poked with biopsy needles, wheeled into operating rooms, and treated with chemotherapy, all for a tumor that would not have caused symptoms, grown bigger, or spread. And let's not forget that medical interventions such as biopsies and chemotherapy come with their own complications such as infection, bleeding, and even death. Also consider that the cost of overdiagnosis is $210 billion a year, according to the Institute of Medicine.

Looking at x-rays and CT scans of my patients, I'd sometimes come across a lump in an area that I wasn't focused on. A patient comes in with a shoulder problem and I'd order an x-ray of the shoulder that would capture part of the lung. And I would see a lump in the lung.

We called those lumps "incidentalomas" and wracked our brains about what to do with them. If a person only had shoulder pain and no chest symptoms, was it worth sending them down a long road of anxiety and biopsies for a lump that wasn't causing problems or may go away on its own?

On the other hand, what if the lump was right on the cusp of being large enough to be considered a potential cancer? Ultimately, it's the doctor's job to empower the patient with information and the patient's right to choose what they want. But these decisions are never as simple as we would like. Have you ever seen the face of a woman after she's told to come back for a chat with the doctor because the mammogram may have detected something or just for a repeat mammogram because the first wasn't clear? It's a harrowing and seemingly long wait till the next appointment.

Critics of studies that show mammograms don't reduce metastatic cancer or cancer deaths have challenged the quality of the mammograms and, in some cases, the study designs. They worry the results will deter women from having breast cancer screening.

This is complicated territory. On the one hand, we all want cancer rates to go down and cancer survival to increase. On the other hand, we don't want women being harmed while we look for early cancers. For the medical profession, it means walking a fine line of advocating for responsible screening while educating about the risks of overdiagnosis and overtreatment.

That's not to say screening is not useful. One study found one-third of the drop in the breast cancer death rate was because of screening. But screening isn't responsible for the biggest reduction in mortality. That was a result of better chemotherapy options to treat the disease, the researchers said.

And again, they identified overdiagnosis as a problem. "Women were more likely to have breast cancer that was overdiagnosed than to have earlier detection of a tumor that was destined to become large," the authors concluded.

All of this has led to disagreement between the leading American medical institutions, none of which can agree on who should get breast screening and when.

The American Cancer Society suggests women with an average risk of developing breast cancer (a one in eight chance over an eighty-year lifetime) get yearly mammograms from ages 45 to 54 then every one to two years after that. Yearly screening with a mammogram should stop when life expectancy is less than ten years. The society says women can get annual screening between ages 40 to 44 years if they choose.

The US Preventive Services Task Force (USPSTF) recommends women begin screening with mammograms at age 50 and continue every other year until age 74. But the American College of Obstetricians and Gynecologists (ACOG) recommends women are offered mammograms every one to two years beginning at age 40 and that screening mammograms should start no later than age 50. Yearly or biennial screening should continue until at least age 75.

The American College of Radiology and the Society for Breast Imaging recommend starting yearly mammograms at age 40 but suggest stopping when life expectancy is estimated to be less than five to seven years. The American College of Physicians says that "if an informed woman requests it," she can have a screening mammogram every two years while in her forties, but doctors should encourage biennial mammograms for women ages 50 to 75. After that age or whenever life expectancy is less than ten years, screening should stop.

If the guidelines don't appear too different, consider this: a woman who chooses to follow the ACOG guidelines could have as many as thirty-four mammograms by age 74 years, which is nearly three times as many mammograms as a woman who follows the USPSTF guidelines.

Where does that leave women? All the guidelines talk about a woman having the right to choose when she begins breast screening, but when even the medical community can't reach consensus, making a choice is difficult.

———————

Guidelines are there to—as the word suggests—guide doctors and they should be a starting point for a discussion, not hard and fast rules about what to do with your body. When making a personal decision about when and how to go about breast cancer screening, take into consideration the following:

Your age: For women in their forties, the chance of being diagnosed with breast cancer is one in sixty-nine. That increases to one in forty-two for women in their fifties and one in twenty-nine for women in their sixties. The medical organizations writing cancer screening guidelines can't agree on when women should start and how often we should have mammograms, but you can consider your current age (and the factors below) in deciding when to start screening.

Family history: The risk of developing breast cancer is impacted by how many of your first-degree relatives have ever been diagnosed with breast cancer (this includes male and female relatives on both your mother's and father's sides). The risk of developing breast cancer is doubled when one first-degree relative has had breast cancer. The risk is tripled if two first-degree relatives had cancer. The risk is higher if the relative was diagnosed before the age of 50.

Genetics: Around one in ten breast cancers are due to mutations inherited from parents. The most common genetic mutations are in the *BRCA1* and *BRCA2* genes, but mutations in some other genes have also been discovered. Talk to your doctor about your need to get tested for these mutations, because it's not appropriate or useful for every woman to have genetic testing.

Your medical history: Women who have had breast cancer are more likely to develop it a second time. Other breast diseases such as lobular carcinoma in situ and atypical hyperplasia are not cancerous but can increase the risk of developing breast cancer. Having radiation to the chest area before the age of 30 or 40 (to treat certain cancers) increases the risk of developing breast cancer. So does being born to a mother who took a medicine called DES while she was pregnant with you. (DES is a hormone that was prescribed between 1940 and 1971 to prevent miscarriage.) Women who took DES themselves are also at a higher risk. Using hormone replacement therapy in menopause can also slightly increase the risk of developing breast cancer depending on which combination of hormones are taken and for how long.

Your reproductive history: Starting periods before the age of 12 and going into menopause after age 55 also raises the risk, because it means you were exposed to hormones for a longer time. Getting pregnant for the first time after the age of 30, never having a full-term pregnancy, and never breast-feeding also increases the risk of developing breast cancer.

Lifestyle: Obesity, a sedentary lifestyle, and drinking more than one alcoholic drink a day can increase the risk of developing breast cancer.

Dense breasts: Women with dense breasts, meaning there's more fibrous tissue and less fatty tissue, have a higher risk of developing breast cancer (it's thought that having dense breast tissue may be linked to higher hormone exposure). The fibrous tissue can also obscure lumps, making it harder to screen using mammograms. You can't tell if you have dense breasts by touching them, but your doctor can tell you after a mammogram. It's not rare—it's thought that up to half of women have dense breasts.

Race: White women are more likely to develop breast cancer than African American, Asian, and Hispanic women, but white women are more likely to live longer past their diagnosis. African American women are twice as likely to develop aggressive cancer or to be diagnosed later and are 42 percent more likely to die from breast cancer than non-Hispanic white women. Some of this has to do with genetics—African American women have a higher risk of *BRCA1* and *BRCA2* mutations than white women—but the later diagnosis and higher death rate is because of institutional racism and inequities in the US health care system.

WHY HAVEN'T YOU MENTIONED BREAST SELF-EXAMINATION?

Because the evidence about whether it's useful or not is . . . conflicting. As if there wasn't enough confusion about breast cancer screening, there's now a debate about whether women should do a monthly self-exam, with some medical organizations advising women do breast exams, others saying not to bother, and some saying there's not enough evidence to make a suggestion either way. Some large studies have shown self-examination didn't help with the early detection of breast cancer but did lead to anxiety through the detection of benign lumps.

On the other hand, women with *BRCA1* or *BRCA2* gene mutations, a previous history of breast cancer, or a family history of breast cancer might benefit from self-exams. In this case it's recommended to do the exam once a month, usually a week after your period ends. Technique is also important, with a move away from starting at the nipple and going in ever larger circles to a vertical technique—according to some experts. There's even a debate about which technique is best.

WHERE TO GO FROM HERE

It's a lot to take in, but going through the list, maybe with the assistance of a relative or friend, can help you determine your risk factors. It's also a helpful starting point for a discussion with your doctor. The decision about if, when, and how often to get mammograms is your decision, and while information can seem overwhelming, it's also empowering.

12

Is it dangerous to be pregnant in America?

first met Shalon Irving in April 2012. We were seated in a huge hotel ball-
room in Atlanta, waiting for the next presenter at the annual Epidemic Intelligence Service Conference to take the stage. Shalon sat in the row ahead
of me, and a mutual friend introduced us as she took a seat. The theme of the
conference that year was inspired by the Hollywood film *Contagion,* starring
Kate Winslet as an EIS officer. We each lugged around a conference handbook
emblazoned with biohazard signs, red tags marked URGENT, and the same
hazy yellow as the *Contagion* movie posters. It was unusual messaging for an
intelligence service that prided itself on training epidemic responders and disease detectives who remained calm at the epicenter of outbreaks and avoided
the roving eyes of reporters and photographers.

I was ten months into my tenure as an officer in the Epidemic Intelligence
Service at the Centers for Disease Control and Prevention, and Shalon was
less than three months away from joining the EIS. The conference was her
introduction to her soon-to-be job and a time for matching with the division

or center that would be her home for the two-year fellowship. Shalon matched with the surveillance branch of the Division of Violence Prevention in the CDC's National Center for Injury Prevention and Control. One of eight Black women in a cohort of eighty-four incoming officers, she would study the health differences between Americans of different races.

At the conference the following year, Shalon gave a talk about food security and high blood pressure among white, Black, and Hispanic people. The next time I heard about Shalon was in an email in 2017 announcing her death. Five years after joining the CDC and three weeks after giving birth to a baby girl, Shalon had died. She was 36 years old.

A Black woman with a PhD, two master's degrees, and a job as lieutenant commander in the US Public Health Service, Shalon died because doctors dismissed her symptoms. In the days after her baby, Soleil, was born, Shalon had a painful lump on her Cesarean-section (C-section) scar, high blood pressure, and a swollen leg, symptoms that were dismissed by health care workers. Shalon's research focused on disparities in health. Precisely the thing that killed her.

Pregnancy and childbirth should be safe around the world and especially in the United States, a high-income country that lauds itself as leader of the "free world." But as pregnancy becomes safer for mother and baby around the world, the opposite is happening in the United States, where pregnancy is becoming more dangerous. Maternal mortality dropped in 157 countries between 2000 and 2013 but went up 27 percent in the United States over a similar time period. Every year, up to 900 American women die from complications of pregnancy and childbirth and up to 63,000 suffer horrifying, preventable complications, including severe bleeding and organ failure. The CDC says 50,000 American women suffer near-death complications of pregnancy every year.

The United States ranks lower than Kazakhstan, Kuwait, and Libya when it comes to keeping pregnant women alive. Black women in America suffer most. Black women are three to four times more likely to die during pregnancy, childbirth, or the months after having a baby than white women.

"The U.S. maternal mortality rate is moving in the wrong direction," said researchers who analyzed maternal mortality in the United States. They published their findings in 2016 in the journal *Obstetrics and Gynecology*. The maternal death rate went up from 18.8 percent in 2000 to 23.8 percent in

2014, they found. California was the only state where things were improving. Texas was so bad that the researchers had to analyze the maternal death rate in that state separately, because it skewed the analysis for the rest of the country. The number of pregnant women and new mothers who died in Texas doubled between 2010 and 2012.

Is health care spending the problem? The United States spends twice as much money on health care compared to other high-income countries but has the worst infant mortality and maternal mortality rates, according to data from a study by researchers at the London School of Economics and Harvard University in 2018.

Comparing the United States with ten high-income countries including Canada, the United Kingdom, Switzerland, and Australia, they found the United States spends 17.8 percent of its gross domestic product on health care, compared to 12.4 percent in Switzerland and less than 10 percent in Australia. The United States spent almost double—$1,443 per person on average—for medicines, compared with $749 per person on average for the other high-income countries in the study.

The United States also spent more on care related to childbirth than any other area of hospitalization, according to an editorial in the journal *Contraception*. The editors called the deaths of mothers in the United States "a human rights failure." The United States spends more than $86 billion per year on child-birth-related care, including spending more money on C-section childbirths than many developed nations.

That last point offers a clue into why more mothers and babies are dying in the United States. The reasons behind the rising maternal mortality rate are complex and intertwined, but too many interventions could be one of the root causes.

One in three American babies enters the world through an incision in the mother's abdomen. The C-section rate increased 60 percent during 1996 to 2011. While the surgery can save lives—for example, when the placenta is blocking the cervix, when labor suddenly slows or stops, or when a baby is breech—the surgery does not come without complications. When there is no medical need for a C-section, the harms of those complications, risks such as infection and bleeding, outweigh the benefits.

But the United States isn't alone in its love of C-sections. The surgery has doubled around the world in less than a generation. In 2000, around one in ten babies was born via C-section. That increased to more than one in five babies born by C-section in 2015.

Another overused intervention in the United States is inducement of labor. One in five pregnant women is given drugs such as oxytocin to increase contractions of the uterus and speed up childbirth. Medications have side effects; in this case, the drugs used to induce labor can cause severe or abnormal contractions that could starve the baby of oxygen, and the mother might have to undergo a C-section. Labor induction also means the uterus is less likely to contract properly after childbirth, which can lead to severe bleeding. The force of contractions can split the uterus along previous scar lines, and in some cases the uterus has to be removed.

Unnecessary interventions are one part of the problem. Many of the causes behind the rising maternal mortality rate are systemic—including racism. Black women are three to four times more likely to die from complications of pregnancy than white women, are less likely to receive the correct pain relief, and are more likely to have serious symptoms ignored.

Education doesn't save Black women's lives on the maternity ward, as evidenced by Shalon's death three weeks after giving birth. Celebrity status and money doesn't help either. In the January 2018 edition of *Vogue* magazine, tennis superstar Serena Williams told her harrowing story of childbirth. She developed a blood clot in her lung the day after giving birth to her first child. Struggling to breathe and aware that she had a medical history of the illness, Williams said health care providers dismissed her. Then her C-section incision split open, possibly because she was gasping for air and coughing.

It's an extension of the racism and misogyny Black women face in office buildings, on public transport, in grocery stores, and on the street, into medical establishments and onto the pages of electronic medical records. Serious symptoms are discounted. Common complications such as blood clots after C-section surgery are not looked for.

Those experiences, in clinics, in grocery stores, everywhere, build up over time to cause a toxic storm of stress that prematurely ages the body. That's according to a theory put forward by Dr. Arline Geronimus, a public health researcher at the University of Michigan. Geronimus was the first to note the association between this lifelong stress, its impact on the body, and the high rates of death among Black babies in America.

She called her theory "weathering."

Weathering can be linked to another phenomenon known as John Henryism, a strategy for coping with the psychological stress of being Black in America, but a coping strategy that causes physical harm and more stress. John Henryism relies on grit, hard work, and the avoidance of support. The term was coined by Professor Sherman James, an epidemiologist studying health differences between Black and white North Carolinians who named his idea after two people: a real life John Henry Martin, a retired Black sharecropper he met in 1978, and John Henry the Black folk hero—who might be based on a real person who lived in the late 1800s.

The John Henry that James met in the seventies was born into a family of sharecroppers in 1907 and worked his way to owner of 75 acres of land in North Carolina by 1947. But he suffered a stomach ulcer so large that nearly half his stomach had to be removed, as well as high blood pressure and arthritis. This was the cost of a Black person working his way to some level of autonomy in America, James concluded. The combination of backbreaking work and structural racism took its toll on the bodies of Black Americans. At their first meeting in the summer of 1978, John Henry Martin told James his arthritis was a consequence of having "pushed too hard in the fields" in the hopes of paying off the mortgage on the farm as soon as he could.

The John Henry of folklore is also known as the steel-driving man, his story told in songs such as Johnny Cash's "Legend of John Henry's Hammer." That John Henry was a formerly enslaved man who was the strongest steel-driver on the Chesapeake & Ohio Railroad—more powerful than the steam-powered drill competing for his role. In a man versus machine showdown, John Henry outdigs the drill but keels over and dies from exhaustion.

The physical and mental strain of fighting against the machine, whether a literal machine or the structurally racist systems that continue today, can be deadly. Geronimus noted that the consequences manifest early in the lives of Black Americans. In 1992 she wrote, "the health of African-American women may begin to deteriorate in early adulthood as a physical consequence of cumulative socioeconomic disadvantage."

This has a negative effect on children. Black American babies are at least twice as likely as white babies to die, a situation far worse than in 1850, when Black people were enslaved and considered property. Now, for every 1,000 Black babies born in the United States, eleven die, compared to fewer than five for every 1,000 white babies. Add up those numbers and you see a harrowing story: every year in America, 4,000 Black babies are born who will never make it to their kindergarten graduation.

When I compared postpregnancy health care protocols between the United States, where I trained as a public health doctor, and the United Kingdom, where I qualified as a doctor and worked as an internist, I found interesting differences. The United Kingdom has national protocols for complications such as post-partum hemorrhage, the United States does not. Women in the United States are less likely to have access to primary care compared to the United Kingdom and other developed nations. There's also poor linkage between maternal care and primary care in the United States.

Across the States, there are big differences in the way pregnancy-related deaths are reviewed. Around half the country doesn't have review boards on maternal mortality, making it hard to understand why women are dying in pregnancy and childbirth.

Some states appear to be hiding data. To stop a problem, you have to understand it, and that requires information. Sounds straightforward, but that's not the case in Texas, where the data public health researchers need are kept secret by the state. If it were available, public health officials could use these data to design and implement interventions that save lives.

"They say they're trying to protect patient privacy, but they could just cross out patient names and any identifiers," said Dr. Robert Gunby, acting chair of the department of obstetrics and gynecology at Baylor University Medical Center.

"We've got to be able to get access to the data and to see why these deaths are occurring and why we're different to California where things are improving."

Texas, with the highest rate of maternal mortality in the United States, lies in stark contrast to California. I used to live in Dallas; it's where I cut my teeth as a newspaper writer at the *Dallas Morning News* and first reported on the crisis of pregnant women and new mothers dying. I now live in California, where I study health communication. My new home is a much safer place to be pregnant.

While more mothers are dying in Texas, fewer mothers are dying in California. The maternal mortality rate in California decreased 30 percent between 2003 and 2014. The experts say that's because "California has made concerted efforts to reduce maternal mortality," including a statewide review of maternal deaths and the use of tool kits to prevent two common causes of maternal deaths: bleeding during delivery and preeclampsia, a pregnancy illness where the woman suffers high blood pressure and potential damage to organs, including the kidneys and liver.

Texas saw a steady rise in the maternal mortality rate from 2000 to 2010 and then a rapid doubling of the death rate within two years: "in the absence of war, natural disaster, or severe economic upheaval, the doubling of a mortality rate within a two-year period in a state with almost 400,000 annual births seems unlikely. A future study will examine Texas data by race-ethnicity and detailed causes of death to better understand this unusual finding," wrote the authors of a study published in *Obstetrics and Gynecology*. They said the lack of available data makes it hard for them to understand what's going on in Texas.

Researchers at Texas Tech asked if the dramatic rise was due to a change in the way the deaths are coded or changes in death certificates. They concluded that wasn't the case.

What did happen over the same period as maternal deaths in Texas were skyrocketing was this: the state's family planning budget was cut by two-thirds in 2011. This led to direct funding cuts of prenatal care clinics, especially those for poor women. The cuts also affected clinics where women could have safe abortions.

Two years later, in 2013, the antiabortion bill HB2 was passed by the Texas legislature. The bill increased the average distance a woman has to travel to get a safe abortion from seventeen miles to seventy miles (the national average is thirty miles). The number of doctors able to provide safe abortions dropped from forty-eight to twenty-eight.

Texas seems to be a hotbed of all the problems afflicting pregnant women across the country. Researchers at Texas Tech looked at the records of 557 Texas women who died during or shortly after pregnancy and discovered bleeding to death, heart attack, and infection were some of the most common causes of death. Of the women who died, one in three died during the first day of hospitalization, the study found. The majority of pregnant women in the study were sick enough to be admitted to the ICU. Gunby said it's a scenario he has witnessed. "Women present late to the hospital so a problem that could have been solved earlier becomes very serious," he said.

Drug overdose was the second-leading cause of maternal death in Texas in 2011 and 2012, according to a report published in July by the Texas Maternal Mortality and Morbidity Task Force. Drug overdoses ranked second only to hypertension, a more commonly seen cause of maternal death around the world. "The majority of these maternal deaths involved licit or illicit prescription opioids. This finding is alarming and may represent an ongoing shift in maternal causes of death," the authors said. "We see that in our clinic," said Gunby. "We have lots of pregnant women who come to the clinic who have overdosed."

And as in the rest of the United States, Black women in Texas are at highest risk of death. Except it's much worse in Texas. About one in ten Texas babies is born to a Black mother, but Black women account for almost a third of all maternal deaths. The report by the Texas Task Force found huge racial disparities in maternal mortality. Hispanic women account for nearly half of all births in Texas and make up a third of maternal deaths. Hispanic women also have a lower rate of severe illness during pregnancy compared with Black women.

Texas did not expand Medicaid to include more poor adults, as encouraged under the Affordable Care Act, and that means more new moms are unable to access care sixty days after delivery, said Gunby. "If they're severely depressed they can't get their antidepressant. If they have hypertension, which is very common and they can develop heart disease from it . . . they won't get treatment," he said.

Broad societal issues such as poverty and a lack of medical insurance are at the heart of the rise in maternal deaths, said Gunby. He set up a program for pregnant women who were otherwise unable to get care. "We were seeing these women who showed up in the emergency room over and over without insurance," he said. "Now we see them two days a week in an after-hours clinic to make sure they get care."

✓ THIS IS IMPORTANT

While it may seem tempting to advise pregnant women to seek prenatal counseling, lose weight, and eat well, what needs to change is policy and what needs to be talked about frankly is structural inequalities and racism in the health care system, which is exactly what Shalon Irving had dedicated her life to fighting.

Shalon died because her very high blood pressure after birth, and bloody discharge and pain from her C-section wound, were dismissed by some health care staff who told her it was nothing. In the email her colleagues received to inform us of her death, we were reminded of Shalon's mission of ending inequality. Her Twitter bio said: "I see inequity wherever it exists, call it by name, and work to eliminate it."

13

The raging statin debate
Should you take a cholesterol-lowering drug?

I f you are over the age of 40, chances are you already pop a cholesterol-lowering pill called a statin. An estimated 32 million Americans take statins—a number equivalent to the combined populations of Texas and Oklahoma. Statins can lower bad cholesterol, known as LDL, by 30 percent and are estimated to prevent thousands of strokes and heart attacks in the United States each year.

But the medicine is not without controversy. In some studies, as many as one-third of people taking statins suffered side effects and half stopped taking the drugs because they had muscle pain, flushing, or confusion. In rare cases, people experience liver damage, memory loss, or a breakdown of muscle tissue. Statins can also increase the risk of diabetes, particularly in women.

The medicine is causing a fight in the medical world, pitching two high-profile journals against one another. On the one side are those who say millions more people should take statins. On the other side are those who argue that statins are overprescribed and that studies highlighting their benefits are often funded by the drug companies that make them.

Guidelines published in 2013 said 56 million Americans aged 40 to 75 were eligible to take statins. But older guidelines said 43 million Americans were eligible. In the United Kingdom, a study published in 2016 said one-third of British adults should be taking statins.

The study looked at thirty years of data and found that if 10,000 people with heart disease take a statin for five years, the drug will prevent heart attacks and strokes in 1,000 people. In terms of side effects, the researchers calculated that if the same number of people took a statin, five would develop muscle aches, one would develop serious breakdown of muscle tissue, fifty to a hundred would develop diabetes, and five to ten would suffer bleeding into the brain over the course of five years.

The study was published in the *Lancet,* the same journal that published a fraudulent study in 1998 that falsely said vaccines cause autism. It took the *Lancet* twelve years to retract the damaging article about the vaccine, and studies show it is still having a negative impact on vaccination rates.

What does the fraudulent vaccine paper have to do with cholesterol? Well, burned by that experience, the *Lancet* editor in chief Richard Horton published the study recommending one in three Brits should be on statins, and in a separate op-ed he argued that research undermining the benefit of statins was harming the public's health.

"We saw in a very painful way the consequences of publishing a paper which had a huge impact on confidence in a safe and effective vaccine," said Horton.

"After publication of disputed research and tendentious opinions about statin use . . . patients already taking statins were more likely to stop their medication," Horton wrote. "Some research papers are more high risk to public health than others."

The research that Horton is referring to questions the use of statins in low-risk people. It was published in a competing medical journal, the *British Medical Journal,* in 2013. In that issue, the *BMJ* ran two papers, both stating that statins do not reduce deaths and that for some, the side effects of statins may outweigh the benefits.

In the United States, current guidelines have moved away from setting target levels of LDL and instead split patients at high risk of heart attack or stroke into four groups:

Group 1: People who already have heart disease.

Group 2: People with an LDL level of 190 mg/dl or higher.

Group 3: People aged 40 to 75 who have type 2 diabetes.

Group 4: People aged 40 to 75 who have a ten-year risk of
            heart disease that is 7.5 percent or higher.

If you fall into groups 1, 2, or 3, you are eligible to take statins. If your doctor used a risk calculator such as the one on the website of the World Health Organization and determined that you fall into group 4, you are also eligible to take a statin. But it's this fourth group that is causing concern for some scientists, since the older guidelines recommended statins for people with a ten-year risk of heart disease of 10 to 20 percent, not a ten-year heart disease risk of 7.5 percent or higher.

Some doctors argue that the new guidelines turn healthy people into patients. For example, people in group 4 may not have any symptoms of heart disease but will be prescribed a pill to take every day for the rest of their lives. That's a type of prevention known in public health as primary prevention. There's also criticism that the heart risk calculator overemphasizes some risk factors while ignoring others, such as family history.

So, should you take a statin? Ask two doctors and you may get two different answers. Throw into the mix a growing body of evidence that says the cholesterol you eat has little impact on the amount of cholesterol in your bloodstream and you have a situation that is confusing—even to experts.

Ongoing studies aim to clarify the situation rather than complicate it. In the meantime, you can check out the WHO's heart risk calculator, study the evidence on both sides of the argument, and have a discussion about the guidelines with your provider.

The statin debate is a reminder that doctors don't have all the answers and that the best health care decisions are made when well-informed people can engage with open-minded doctors.

14

Does aspirin prevent cancer?

You've probably heard that for some people taking a small dose of aspirin every day can help prevent heart attacks and strokes. You may be one of the millions of people around the world who uses aspirin for this reason. Since the landmark Physicians' Health Study that began in 1982, we've known that low-dose aspirin, also known as baby aspirin, referring to a dose between 75 mg and 150 mg, can decrease the risk of a first heart attack by 44 percent. (The regular dose taken for aches and pains is 325 mg.)

Doctors have been prescribing aspirin to prevent heart attacks and strokes ever since that study. But there's new evidence that possibly the most researched medicine on the planet could help prevent and lower the risk of death from certain cancers.

When scientists studied people who were taking aspirin to prevent heart attacks and stroke, they found an interesting difference between those who took aspirin regularly and those who didn't. According to some follow-up studies, those taking regular aspirin had a lower risk of cancer and death from cancer.

In a study of more than half a million people published in the *New England Journal of Medicine* in 1991, aspirin use at least sixteen times per month was associated with a 40 percent lower risk of death from colon cancer over a six-year period.

More recently, in a 2017 study at Harvard Medical School, researchers looked at more than 86,000 women who were part of the Nurses' Health Study and 43,000 men who were part of the Health Professionals Follow-Up Study between the 1980s and 2012.

Over three decades, more than 8,200 women and more than 4,500 men in the study died of cancer but aspirin use was associated with a lower risk of death, compared with those who didn't use aspirin regularly. Overall, aspirin use was associated with a 7 percent lower risk of death from cancer for women and 15 percent lower risk of death from cancer for men.

The link with colorectal cancer was especially apparent. Regular aspirin use was associated with a 30 percent lower risk of dying from colorectal cancer in men and women and an 11 percent lower risk of death from breast cancer in women.

The use of the word *associated* is important here. Observational studies like these can't prove that one thing causes another. But they can show links between two things and pave the way to more solid studies.

In observational studies such as case-controlled and cohort studies, researchers look at groups of people, in this case, some taking aspirin regularly and others not taking it regularly or not taking it at all, and they make comparisons between the groups. Like all studies, observational studies are subject to bias. In both of these studies, participants were asked to self-report if they took aspirin regularly, which can be an inaccurate way of collecting data (people forget things, they mistake aspirin for Tylenol, or they straight up lie).

But the association between lower risk of cancer and aspirin use could be because of some other factor, not the aspirin. Regular use of aspirin could be a surrogate for a healthier lifestyle. People taking aspirin may be generally more health conscious and have fewer risk factors for cancer such as obesity and smoking.

Midway up the pyramid of evidence, above case-controlled and cohort studies, are randomized controlled trials, or RCTs. These are the gold standard of clinical studies. They're designed to limit bias as much as is humanly possible by randomly allocating participants to groups. Some groups will take regular aspirin, other groups might take a different treatment, and others might take a placebo. Ideally, the study will be "blind" and no one will know which group they are in or which treatment they are taking—not even the health care workers handing out the pills. The idea is to prevent personal beliefs about a particular treatment from influencing the study.

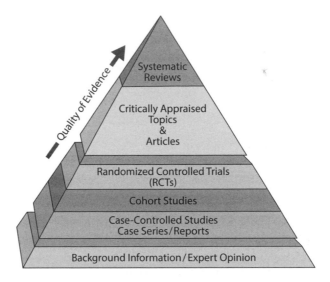

Ask, how strong is the evidence? All studies are not equal. The pyramid of evidence-based medicine is a hierarchy of the quality of different types of evidence.

At least four RCTs and a meta-analysis of RCTs, have shown that in patients with a history of colorectal cancer, aspirin lowers the short-term risk of the cancer coming back. But it takes a while for this effect to show. In fact, low-dose aspirin has to be taken every day for five to ten years before the cancer prevention benefits show.

ASPIRIN AND METASTATIC CANCER

Sometimes researchers group lots of observational studies together, combine the data, and analyze them in what's known as a meta-analysis. In a 2012 meta-analysis of observational studies of aspirin and cancer, researchers looked at studies published between 1950 and 2011 and found that regular aspirin use was associated with a lower risk of developing certain cancers and a lower risk of an existing cancer spreading throughout the body.

What does aspirin have to do with metastatic cancer? It turns out that metastatic cancer, where cancer cells travel through the body and cause secondary tumors, co-opt platelets for the cancer's advantage. Platelets, responsible for helping blood to clot, can form a protective cloak around cancer cells, sneak them into blood vessels, and help them spread to distant parts of the body. Once the cancer cells have spread, they instruct platelets to make chemicals that spur the growth of new blood vessels. The new blood vessels feed the new tumor. Aspirin is an antiplatelet drug. It blocks the formation of a chemical called thromboxane A2, which platelets need if they want to clump together.

Aspirin also targets DNA. Platelets don't contain DNA, but aspirin seems to switch off groups of genes in other blood cells, which gives rise to platelets so they can't aggregate and cloak errant cancer cells.

Yet, not everyone is susceptible to aspirin's antimetastatic effects. Scientists are devising genetic tests to determine if a person is susceptible or if it's not worth the risk of taking aspirin. The goal is to give aspirin to those who benefit but not prescribe it to those who would see no effects, because adverse events caused by aspirin include bleeding.

Studies on aspirin and its effect on metastatic cancer are in the early stages. As scientists learn more, they're uncovering new ways in which aspirin works.

CONTRADICTORY GUIDANCE

Should you take aspirin to prevent cancer? The answer depends on which medical organization you ask. The US Preventive Services Task Force (USPSTF) in 2016 recommended low-dose aspirin to prevent cardiovascular disease and colorectal cancer in adults aged 50 to 59 years, but only if they meet the following criteria: a person who is likely to live at least another ten years and is willing to take low-dose aspirin every day for that time, has at least a 10 percent risk of a heart attack or stroke in that decade, and is not at increased risk for bleeding.

Since aspirin interferes with platelets and clotting, one of its most dangerous side effects is bleeding in the stomach, brain, and elsewhere. People with stomach ulcers or on certain medications that interact with aspirin are at the highest risk of bleeding. This is an important side effect that has to be taken into consideration when weighing the risks and benefits of long-term aspirin use. (Less serious side effects of aspirin include indigestion, nausea, and heartburn.)

For adults aged 60 to 69 years, the USPSTF says the decision to start low-dose aspirin is an individual one. It says there is not enough evidence to offer guidance for adults younger than 50 years or older than 70.

By suggesting that healthy people take a medicine to prevent an illness that they don't have, the USPSTF is recommending a type of prevention called primary prevention. (Secondary prevention is lessening the impact of a disease that already exists, such as when a person who has had a stroke takes aspirin every day to prevent a second stroke.)

Here's where other agencies disagree with the USPSTF. The Food and Drug Administration does not recommend aspirin for primary prevention. Nor does the European Society of Cardiology.

While doctors are still debating who should take aspirin, its popularity is on the rise. Between 2005 and 2010, there was a 57 percent increase in the regular use of aspirin among Americans. And even before the USPSTF published its aspirin and cancer guidelines in 2016, people had read the studies (and the sometimes misleading headlines) and started taking aspirin in the hopes of preventing cancer. Almost a fifth of Americans taking aspirin regularly said they were doing so for cancer prevention, according to one study.

If you're aged 50 to 59 you can choose to go with the USPSTF's guidelines, talk to your doctor to calculate your ten-year heart attack and stroke risk (or use an online calculator to do the same), and go from there. Even then, your doctor may or may not agree with the Task Force's recommendations. For everyone else, the guidance is even more blurry. But with close to 1,000 clinical trials involving aspirin each year, that guidance could become clearer, or we'll discover yet more potential benefits of aspirin.

15

Did the maker of aspirin test medicines in Nazi concentration camps?

One of the most popular medicines in the world, taken by upward of 40 million Americans a day, has a little-known Nazi connection. Some survivors of Auschwitz and other Holocaust concentration camps still refuse to take any medicines made by the drug company Bayer because of the aspirin manufacturer's connection with Adolf Hitler's quest to wipe out Jewish people.

Before it became entangled with the horrors of the Holocaust, the herbal remedy that inspired aspirin was an ancient Egyptian treatment for ear infections, among other things.

Here's a pre–Nazi era primer on aspirin.

The herbal remedy that inspired aspirin is mentioned in the oldest medical text in history, the Ebers Papyrus, written in the sixteenth century before Christ. In a series of hieroglyphs the Ebers Papyrus says: *if the ear opening discharges you should prepare a powder to dry the wound with the juice of acacia, juice of Zizyphus, cumin and a hint of willow.*

Much later, an eighteenth-century Englishman decided to taste a piece of wood, specifically willow bark. Reverend Edward Stone noticed the bark tasted bitter, and that reminded him of a different bark that was used to help treat fevers. He wondered if willow bark would be an effective treatment for what was then known as ague, meaning an illness with bouts of shivering.

Stone's idea was based on the doctrine of signatures, a belief that wherever there is the cause of disease, the cure is close by, like using the smooth dock leaves on a nettle plant to relieve the nettles' sting. Back in eighteenth-century England, fevers were thought to attack in cool, damp areas like riverbanks, exactly the place where willow trees grow. Following the doctrine of signatures, Reverend Stone picked some willow bark, dried it for months next to an oven, ground the wood into powder, and gave it to people suffering fevers.

It took over a hundred years for the idea to catch on in the Western world and only after a Scottish doctor did a study showing the active ingredient in willow bark, salicylic acid, really did alleviate fevers. But there was a problem. Once they knew it worked, they needed to be able to mass produce salicylic acid, and they weren't keen on the idea of stripping thousands of willow trees and gathering tons of bark.

This is where the German company Bayer enters the picture, or as it was known then, Farbenfabriken vorm. Friedr. Bayer & Co. In the late 1800s, what is now Bayer was making synthetic dyes. But by the end of that century it branched into making medicines. In 1897, a Bayer scientist synthesized a stable form of acetylsalicylic acid and in 1899, the company launched the drug for the first time under the trade name Aspirin. By 1919, Bayer was generating around 30 percent of its global sales from aspirin in the United States.

The tale of who first synthesized aspirin is telling of the next phase of the drug's history. In the footnotes of a book published in 1934, Bayer scientist Felix Hoffmann took credit for the discovery. But that specific date raised suspicions for a Scottish scientist who was digging through Bayer's records in the late 1990s.

Walter Sneader, a medicinal chemist at the University of Strathclyde in Scotland, saw Hoffmann's notes on his so-called discovery and wasn't convinced. "The date of 1934 was intriguing," he said to reporters. "The Nazis had just come to power. They had already taken steps to get Jews out of professions.

Anti-Semitism was sweeping Germany. That's when Hoffmann's story first appeared."

Sneader found laboratory notebooks that revealed aspirin was first synthesized by Hoffmann's colleague, Arthur Eichengrün, a German Jew. "[Hoffmann] was just a technician," he said. "It's the same today. If I was working with the world's greatest chemist and he told me what to synthesize, he would get the credit for what was produced, not me."

To this day, the Bayer Group's Corporate History department cites Hoffmann as the first chemist to synthesize the drug even though evidence points to Eichengrün first synthesizing aspirin in a laboratory. It seems Eichengrün was denied credit because he was Jewish.

But that's not why some Jewish people refuse to take aspirin.

By the time Hoffmann published his book in the 1930s, Bayer's parent company, Bayer A.G., had merged with I.G. Farben, the most powerful corporate cartel in Germany. It was also the largest commercial profiteer from the Second World War. Some historians say Hitler's quest to kill millions of Jews, Gypsies, and gay people couldn't have happened without the chemical help of I.G. Farben and its companies.

The conglomerate was formed of groups including Hoechst, BASF, Bayer, and Degesch. It was Degesch that made Zyklon B, the gas used to kill prisoners in Nazi concentration camps, doubling the company's profits. It wasn't I.G. Farben's first foray into gas warfare: in the First World War, it supplied the chlorine gas used to kill thousands of French troops in the trenches.

In his book, *The Crime and Punishment of I.G. Farben,* Joseph Borkin describes how I.G. Farben spearheaded the use of Jewish slave labor to build I.G. Auschwitz, the largest plant in the I.G. system. More than 300,000 Auschwitz prisoners were forced to build the plant, at least 25,000 of them were worked to death.

Survivors of the Nazi concentration camps recall doctors force feeding them pills and injecting them with chemicals. Zoe Polanska was 13 years old when she was experimented on in Auschwitz. Eyewitnesses say the doctors who tested drugs on her were working for Bayer.

Zoe lives in Scotland and is demanding Bayer give her compensation and an apology. She was featured in a BBC documentary in 2003 where she spoke about the experiments she endured, which she believes left her battling cancer in her seventies. Zoe said the medicines Bayer tested on her were birth control drugs.

"I still find it difficult to take aspirin," Zoe said in the BBC documentary. "I remember one of the SS doctors holding my jaw open and forcing pills down my throat. I'm still very wary of men wearing white coats."

In 1986, Zoe published a book, *Yalta Victim*, about her family's story from the Soviet Union to Germany and then to Scotland. She recounted seeing the infamous Nazi doctor Josef Mengele experimenting on twins. The children's faces were "shriveled up like old prunes," she said. "Their bushy eyebrows indicated a long stay and some of them had huge pregnant bellies."

Eva Mozes Kor was one of those girls. She survived the medical experiments of Dr. Mengele in Auschwitz and lived most of her life in the United States. "They would give me injections . . . after one of those injections I became very ill. The rumor at the camp was that anyone taken to the hospital would never come back." It wasn't until the 1990s that Kor learned that Bayer was in bed with the Nazis. Eva died in 2019 aged 85.

When the BBC documentary featuring Zoe's story aired in 2003, Bayer issued a statement claiming the company did not exist at the time of the Second World War. "Between 1925 and 1952, no company named Bayer existed, neither as a subsidiary of IG Farben nor as any other legal entity," a Bayer spokesperson told the BBC. "Bayer has worked in good faith with the German government to establish a fund to help those who have suffered. The company's contribution to this fund amounted to more than £40 million."

Eva, who survived medical experimentation in Auschwitz, refuses to take aspirin or any other medicine made by Bayer. "I really won't support them. I don't think they deserve my support."

Zoe died in 2017 at the age of 89. She was unable ever to have children, a result of electric shocks delivered to her ovaries by Nazi doctors, she said, and she had suffered a long battle with cancer. The German government eventually conceded to her requests for compensation. In 2004, it gave her approximately $2,500.

16

Does the birth control pill cause depression?

I walked into the newsroom one morning in 2016 to find a nervous reporter waiting at my desk. "Is it true?" she whispered. "Could my birth control make me suicidal?" She was in her twenties and had been taking the pill for years, but on her drive to work she'd heard two news reports that said the pill could cause depression and even suicide. She was freaked out and wondering if she should stop taking the pill immediately.

The news reports were based on a study published in the American Medical Association's *JAMA Psychiatry*. But the study design means it cannot determine if the pill causes depression or suicide. I pulled up the paper on my computer as my colleague read over my shoulder and I read out loud the parts that concerned me. "The researchers even say it," I said, scrolling to the end of the paper. "They say it's not possible to say the pill is the cause of these problems." But that hadn't stopped some reporters from stating that birth control causes depression, which led to panic among some women who use the pill. It's part of a pattern: studies not designed to determine causality were reported on as if they have in fact found the cause of some illness.

The study itself is not without flaws but, let's face it, studies are rarely perfect.

Overall, it does a pretty good job of looking at a large group of women over an average of six years and trying to advance an important area of research about depression and hormonal contraception.

The researchers found that each year, 2.2 percent of women using hormonal birth control were likely to start using an antidepressant, compared to 1.7 percent of women not using hormonal birth control. When it came to a diagnosis of depression, 0.3 percent of women using hormonal birth control were diagnosed, compared with 0.28 percent of non-users.

These are not big differences, but you wouldn't know that from looking at the media coverage. Before we look at the news reports, let's break down the study.

The researchers in Denmark looked at the records of 1,061,997 women ages 15 to 34 from 1995 to 2013. They analyzed the data to see if use of hormonal contraception was associated with using an antidepressant and diagnosis of depression at a psychiatric hospital.

Roughly half of the women were current or recent users of hormonal contraception, including the oral contraceptive pill, patch, vaginal ring, implant, injection, or intrauterine system (sometimes known as the hormonal coil). The remaining women did not use any hormonal contraception.

POOR CHOICE OF CONTROL GROUP

This is where the problems begin. Comparing women who use hormonal contraception with those who don't use it isn't ideal. There can be big differences between these two groups of women in terms of their access to medical care and willingness to take medications.

For example, a woman who takes the pill is likely to have a doctor who gives her the prescription for birth control as well as a routine where she pops a pill on a daily basis. Compare that to a woman who doesn't take the pill. She may not be registered with a doctor or she may not see a doctor regularly and may be less willing to take medication.

What epidemiologists worry about is that any variation in the rate of depression between the two groups of women could be explained by differences like these as opposed to hormonal contraception. And bear in mind, one of the key outcomes the study authors were looking at was use of an antidepressant—a medicine that has to be prescribed by a doctor and one that someone averse to popping pills may not be willing to take.

Choosing a control group is tough, but the researchers could have picked a better comparison group. Chelsea Polis, an epidemiologist at the Guttmacher Institute in New York, an organization that researches reproductive health and contraception, said comparison with women who use nonhormonal contraception, such as the copper coil, would have been a better choice and provided more information.

Women who use the copper coil, while not being exposed to hormones like estrogen and progesterone, still use some form of contraception and have a relationship with a physician. In the past, studies comparing women who take the pill to women who use the copper coil found women on the pill were not more likely to have a loss of sexual desire.

ANTIDEPRESSANTS ARE PRESCRIBED FOR A BUNCH OF THINGS OTHER THAN DEPRESSION

The researchers found that women using hormonal contraception were more likely to be prescribed an antidepressant, compared to women who did not use hormonal birth control. But about half of all people taking an antidepressant are taking it for something other than depression. Antidepressants can be prescribed to treat pain, sleeping problems, ADHD, migraine, and problems of the digestive and urinary tracts.

WOMEN EXCLUDED FROM THE STUDY

When you're looking at a study to decide whether it's a good one, it's helpful to look at who the researchers included in the study and who was left out. In this case, women were excluded during pregnancy and for six months after having a baby. The researchers did this "to reduce the influence of post-partum depression," they said.

But Polis is concerned that this could skew the study findings. "Women who are not using hormonal contraception are likely to become pregnant more often and to have more unintentional pregnancies," she said. "So you would think they would be more likely to face post-partum depression or other types of depression around the time of pregnancy, particularly if they were dealing with an unintentional pregnancy."

Polis said she would have liked an additional analysis that didn't exclude women during this time "because it makes 'invisible' any depression that may result from unintended pregnancy or from post-partum depression. Including this could provide a fuller picture for women who need to consider various potential causes of depression in their day-to-day lives."

Those are some flaws of the study. Now on to mistakes made by reporters writing about it.

The study found that women who used hormonal contraception were more likely to get a prescription for an antidepressant or receive a diagnosis of depression. Some news outlets reported an 80 percent increase in depression among women who used these contraceptives. But the 80 percent figure was specific to women ages 15 to 19 who were specifically using the combined oral contraceptive pill.

To communicate the overall risk of depression for women using the combined oral contraceptive pill, it's more accurate to say that taking it was associated with a 10 percent increased risk of being diagnosed with depression.

This may or may not be an acceptable risk for women who take the pill (I'm fine with it, having looked at the study and seen its flaws), but inaccurate media reports could sway a woman's decision and make her abruptly stop taking birth control.

In the study, the forms of contraception associated with the biggest increases in the risk of depression or taking an antidepressant were those that contained only the hormone progestin. The biggest increases were seen in women 15 to 19, and women of that age "are more susceptible to risk factors for depression," the authors write.

Some journalists were picky about which risk estimates they chose to include in their news stories. Many chose to include relative risk, which tells you how more or less likely a disease occurs in one group compared to another. Relative risk does not tell you the actual likelihood that something will happen to you.

A useful way of explaining risk is to explain the absolute risk, and I'm not sure why many journalists shy away from doing this. (One expert was told by a reporter that it was tricky and there wasn't enough space in the article to explain absolute risk. I think this is a disservice to the public, since absolute risk is a helpful way to understand your actual risk of developing a disease.)

While the relative risk can sound high (an 80 percent increase in depression!) the likelihood of depression occurring in the first place is really low. In this study, for instance, I calculated that for every 300 women who use hormonal contraception, an additional one woman will use an antidepressant.

Again, that may or may not be an acceptable number for you (I won't be cancelling my prescription anytime soon), but what is unacceptable to me is the way this study has been misreported. We all deserve accurate reporting on scientific studies so we can make fact-based decisions about our bodies and the pills we take.

17

Do vitamin D supplements protect against obesity, cancer, and pneumonia?

T he vitamin D supplement industry is a multimillion-dollar business. Although vitamin D is a popular dietary supplement, it's hotly debated whether people without a deficiency should take it on a regular basis. Many people choose to take it because of purported health claims that vitamin D protects against obesity, pneumonia, even cancer.

The sunshine vitamin—so called because the sun's rays convert cholesterol into vitamin D in our skin—is important for bone development and helping the body maintain the right amounts of calcium and phosphorus.

We get vitamin D through the sun and through some foods. It's present in egg yolks, oily fish, and cheese but in small amounts. Some countries, such as Sweden, Finland, and the United States, fortify foods with vitamin D3, and there have been calls to do the same in other places, such as the United Kingdom.

But claims that the sunshine vitamin wards off cancer were hype. Celebratory headlines announcing vitamin D prevents colorectal cancer were generated from a 2018 analysis of seventeen international studies including nearly 6,000 cancer patients. The study found a 31 percent higher risk of developing colorectal cancer over five and a half years in people who were deficient in vitamin D. Higher amounts of vitamin D in the blood were associated with a 22 percent lower risk of developing colorectal cancer.

This was an important study because it was building on previous research that had been frustratingly inconclusive. Scientists in the past had used smaller groups of patients and controls and all sorts of vitamin D tests, which made it difficult to make comparisons.

But this study was important for another reason as well. The scientists, some of the most respected vitamin D experts in the world, were specifically saying that vitamin D "concentrations above bone health sufficiency" were associated with a lower risk of colorectal cancer.

That part has the potential to change the way we prescribe and recommend vitamin D supplements and the doses we suggest. The study authors say in the *Journal of the National Cancer Institute* that the amount of vitamin D needed to protect against cancer could be higher than the amount currently recommended by the Institute of Medicine in the United States.

The lifetime risk of colorectal cancer is 4.5 percent for men and 4.2 percent for women. Keep that in mind when considering the risk reduction stated in this study and when deciding if you want to take vitamin D supplements to boost your levels beyond what is needed for healthy bones. Especially because, as with any medicine, there are side effects.

There could be a confounding factor at play. Confounding factors are things that make it appear as though two things are linked. Say a study finds that donut eaters are more likely to get lung cancer. But then it turns out that people who eat donuts (I'm just making this up) are more likely to eat the donut while smoking a cigarette. Well, the true link is between the cigarettes and the lung cancer, and the donut was masquerading as an annoying confounder. You may have heard "murder rates are higher when ice-cream sales are higher." It's unlikely that murderous thoughts are fueled by Cherry Garcia and more likely that murder rates are higher in the summer, when more people are out and interacting with one another. Weather is the confounder.

In the case of this study, what if people with more vitamin D in their blood have different diets and lifestyles compared to people with lower vitamin D levels? What if those factors explain why they have a lower risk of developing cancer? The authors don't get into this, but they do remind us that vitamin D supplements are not recommended for colorectal cancer prevention.

What about childhood obesity? Also in 2018, researchers in Greece said obese children who took a weekly vitamin D supplement every week for a year had a lower body mass index and a lower fat mass compared to obese children who did not take the supplement. But the study size was small—232 children, of whom 117 took a weekly dose of vitamin D—and the authors don't tell us how much fat they lost or how much their BMI dropped.

The researchers also didn't take into account what foods the children ate and how much exercise they had. A year earlier, Polish scientists published their protocol for an ongoing study looking at the effects of vitamin D in obese children enrolled in a weight-loss program.

Many obese children have lower than usual vitamin D levels, possibly because of an unbalanced diet and not enough time playing in the sun. Because of this, and because the vitamin is thought to affect insulin sensitivity in overweight children, the researchers enrolled more than 1,600 obese schoolchildren and gave one group daily vitamin D supplements as well as regular visits with a dietician and physical education specialist. The other group received the same interventions but not vitamin D. While the results of this study haven't been published yet, the study design hopes to offer more comprehensive data on the effects of vitamin D on obesity.

A 2017 study claiming vitamin D prevented pneumonia generated a spate of exciting headlines. But the news stories mostly ignored the study's weaknesses. Researchers at Queen Mary University of London analyzed twenty-five studies looking at the effectiveness of vitamin D in preventing respiratory tract infections. In all, these studies included 11,321 people from a few months of age to 95 years.

Many news stories reported that the number of people who got a chest infection was 12 percent lower in the group taking a vitamin D supplement. What they didn't include was the overall absolute risk reduction—the actual reduction—which was much lower, only 2 to 3 percent. Absolute risk is a helpful way of showing the real magnitude of benefit, but it's often left out of the news.

Another useful way of looking at numbers from studies like this one is how many people would need to take vitamin D for one chest infection to be prevented. The answer in this case is thirty-three. If looking only at people who already had very low levels of vitamin D in their body to begin with, four people would need to take the supplement to prevent one chest infection. Those numbers can help you decide if you think it's worthwhile to take the supplement.

In the study published in the *British Medical Journal,* the researchers went as far as to say that their study "supports the introduction of public health measures such as food fortification to improve vitamin D status."

But in an editorial in the same journal, researchers at the University of Oxford said "there is no evidence that supplementation with vitamin D leads to a reduction in the incidence of acute respiratory tract infections. The data therefore do not support recommendations for population-wide supplementation with vitamin D to prevent acute respiratory tract infections."

Here are some of the study's weaknesses: The researchers didn't look at people according to race, an important factor in vitamin D research, since people with darker skin are more likely to have lower levels of vitamin D. They used a technique called subgroup analysis to look at people of different ages. This type of analysis may have given more dramatic numbers overall. But looking carefully at the different subgroups, the group most likely to have a lower chance of chest infections while taking vitamin D is between 1 and 16 years old. So don't believe the headlines claiming vitamin D supplements are as useful as the flu shot.

Despite this, doctors seem to be prescribing vitamin D in ever larger amounts. And not just to people who have a bona fide deficiency. "Clinical enthusiasm for supplemental vitamin D has outpaced available evidence on its effectiveness," wrote doctors JoAnn E. Manson and Shari S. Bassuk in a 2015 commentary in the *Journal of the American Medical Association.*

Vitamin D blood tests increased eighty-three-fold from 2000 to 2010 in Medicare beneficiaries. Overscreening for vitamin D deficiency is a problem because oftentimes the labs sending back the results report normal levels as insufficient. That's when prescriptions get printed.

But there are side effects. You should be consuming 600 international units of vitamin D a day if you are between the ages of 1 and 70, and 800 international units a day if you're over 71, according to the Institute of Medicine.

You are considered deficient if your blood vitamin D levels are 25 nmol/L or less. But that doesn't mean you need to take vitamin D every day, unless your doctor says so. The Food and Drug Administration says, "Vitamin D is not required in daily dietary intake." That's because the vitamin can be stored in the liver and used when your supplies run low.

Most of us get the right amount of vitamin D through sun exposure and food. If you really are deficient, you may need to take a supplement, but take too much vitamin D and you can suffer a spike in blood calcium levels, which can cause kidney stones, calcification of blood vessels, even heart disease.

The only patients for whom there is evidence that vitamin D supplementation is needed on a regular basis are those at high risk of osteomalacia, a condition where the bones are weakened.

There are exciting discoveries being made about vitamin D and its functions in the body. But it's not proven to prevent cancer, obesity, or pneumonia, and too much of a good thing can be bad.

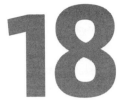

Will fish oil supplements prevent heart disease or give you cancer?

Nearly one in ten Americans uses a fish oil supplement regularly, making it one of the most popular supplements in the United States, say researchers at the National Center for Health Statistics. Americans spend more than $1 billion each year on fish oil.

Many hope the supplements will improve joint health, sharpen the mind, and prevent heart disease and strokes. My mum used to buy fish oil capsules in bulk the months before my high school exams. But data about the health benefits of fish oils are inconsistent and often inconclusive. Sorry, mum.

Fish oils contain two types of omega-3 fatty acids called EPA and DHA (eicosapentaenoic acid and docosahexaenoic acid, respectively). Our bodies can't make these fatty acids, so we have to consume them. Good sources of EPA and DHA are oily fish such as mackerel, herring, and sardines. Some nonanimal foods, such as pumpkin seeds and walnuts, contain a different kind of omega-3 fatty acid, alpha-linoleic acid, which the body converts to DHA and EPA. These fatty acids are transformed by the body into anti-inflammatory chemicals called resolvins.

Omega-3 fatty acids have been touted as preventing heart disease since at least the 1970s, when researchers postulated that Inuit in Canada and Alaska had lower rates of heart disease because they ate a diet rich in fish. That theory was later debunked, and researchers said the Inuit probably have more heart disease than the earlier scientists accounted for.

But claims about fish oil supplements have persisted. The data, however, are unclear. I read through more than thirty studies on fish oils published in the last eight years and found only two that showed the supplements were better than placebos at improving the health of those who took them.

There is some evidence that oily fish and fish oil supplements may ease the pain and swelling of rheumatoid arthritis. One study found that users had less joint pain in the morning and reported that their joints felt less tender. But many studies looking at the effects on rheumatoid arthritis were small and involved users taking multiple supplements. That made it hard to determine if it was the fish oil or something else making them feel less stiff.

Other studies looked at the effect of fish oils on blood pressure. While some reported the supplements did lower blood pressure, these were small studies and not convincing. Other studies found that fish oils had no impact on blood pressure.

There is better evidence that fish oils lower triglyceride levels. Triglycerides are our main form of fat and the type of fat we think about when we talk about fat hips and bellies. But some of the studies claiming fish oils lower triglycerides relied on high doses—up to 4 grams per day—and relied on combining fish oils with other medicines such as statins. Prescription fish oil supplements containing high doses of omega-3 fatty acids have been approved by the Food and Drug Administration, but they can cause serious side effects such as prolonged bleeding.

After a safety review of fish oils in 1997, the FDA said that people should take no more than 3 grams of EPA and DHA per day. Side effects of taking fish oils at high doses range from the annoying—nausea and a fishy burp—to the dangerous—prolonged bleeding caused by a disruption in the clotting system.

Those with risk factors for heart disease and stroke may be disappointed to learn that a study by Italian scientists found fish oils did not prevent these illnesses. More than 12,000 patients were tracked in a study published in 2013.

Half of the study participants received fatty acid supplements, while the rest were given a placebo. Ultimately, those given supplements did not fare better than those given olive oil, which served as the placebo. But this is a very strange choice for a placebo, given that there is some evidence that the fats in olive oil could also lower the risk of heart disease.

In November 2018, the *New England Journal of Medicine* published long-awaited results from fish oil studies including nearly 26,000 people. These adults who were healthy, over the age of 50, and had no history of heart disease or cancer, took either a gram of fish oil or placebo. Some groups were also given vitamin D. After five years, the scientists did not see any overall benefit in those taking the fish oil supplement but did find a lower incidence of heart attack and death from heart attack in people who took fish oil. The incidence of heart attack and fatal heart attacks was reduced by 28 percent in those taking the fish oil supplement, compared to people taking placebo. One-fifth of the study participants were Black, and this group saw a 77 percent decrease in heart attacks and fatal heart attack incidence.

But there's a caveat. Trials are designed with two things in mind: primary endpoints and secondary endpoints. A primary endpoint is the question the trial is optimally designed to answer. It's the main focus of the trial, and the trial is powered and participants randomized for this outcome. Secondary endpoints are other events of interest that the study is not optimally designed to assess. Analysis of secondary endpoints must be done with caution, and in the case of this study, the reduced incidence of heart attacks and fatal heart attacks was a secondary endpoint. The authors said it themselves: "The secondary end points will undoubtedly draw attention. It will be tempting to note the lower incidence of myocardial infarction and of death from myocardial infarction with n-3 fatty acids than with placebo . . . However, these 'positive' results need to be interpreted with caution." They go on to say that these effects have not been consistently seen in other large trials comparing fish oil supplements to placebo.

It looks like we shouldn't be rushing to the store to buy fish oil supplements. And anyway, couldn't we just eat more fish instead of popping pills? After expressing caution over their study results, the scientists call out the medical establishment (particularly the American Heart Association) for writing guidelines recommending omega-3 fatty acids for the prevention of heart disease on "the basis of that one trial," referring to an Italian study published in the 1990s.

There was a knowledge gap about fish oils, they said, and their new study had filled that gap and "convincingly shown that the use of [omega-3] fatty acids is not effective in preventing the combined end point of myocardial infarction, stroke, or death from cardiovascular causes in unselected patients." The findings were consistent with earlier data showing the supplements also had no impact on preventing heart disease in diabetics.

In the past few years, research has emerged showing that fish oils may increase the risk of prostate cancer. In 2013, researchers at the Fred Hutchinson Cancer Research Center in Seattle found that people who take high-dose fish oil supplements or eat a lot of oily fish had a 43 percent increased risk for prostate cancer and a 71 percent increased risk for aggressive prostate cancer.

But even that finding is inconsistent with other studies. In 2017, scientists in Canada published a systematic review of forty-four studies looking at fish oil supplements. They concluded that the "current evidence is insufficient to suggest a relationship between fish-derived omega-3 fatty acid and risk of [prostate cancer]." They suggested that more research is needed.

So, should you take a fish supplement? The American Heart Association recommends eating two servings of oily fish a week. A serving is 3.5 ounces of cooked fish or approximately three-quarters of a cup of flaked fish. Research shows that most Americans eat less than this and opt for fish such as shrimp and canned tuna, which contain fewer omega-3 fatty acids than fish such as mackerel and salmon.

For those with heart disease, the AHA recommends 1 gram of omega-3 fatty acids per day and 2 to 4 grams of fish oil for those with high levels of triglycerides. Always tell your doctor about dietary supplements. Fish oils can interact with the blood-thinning medicine warfarin (also known as Coumadin). Pregnant women should eat no more than 8 ounces of albacore tuna per month and avoid fish high in mercury, including king mackerel and swordfish.

19

Are heartburn medicines linked to a serious gut infection?

The pills you take to control heartburn and suppress stomach acid may be linked to an increased risk of a serious gut infection. A study published in *JAMA Internal Medicine* in 2017 reports that people who take common prescription and over-the-counter indigestion medicines such as Prilosec and Zantac are at risk of repeat infection with the bacteria *Clostridium difficile*.

C. difficile can cause severe swelling of the colon. Symptoms range from mild diarrhea lasting a few days to life-threatening bleeding and leaking of the gut. Previous studies have shown that one class of medicines known as proton pump inhibitors, which are used to suppress stomach acid, can increase risk of a first episode of *C. difficile* infection. Proton pump inhibitors include medicines such as Prevacid, Prilosec, and Nexium, and this class of medicines has also been linked to pneumonia, kidney disease, vitamin B12 deficiency, and fractures related to thinning of the bone possibly caused by malabsorption of calcium.

The new study adds that another class of indigestion medicines called H2 blockers can also increase risk of infection with *C. difficile*. H2 blockers include

Pepcid, Zantac, and Tagamet. Researchers at the Mayo Clinic in Rochester, Minnesota, analyzed data from sixteen older studies, which included 7,703 patients who suffered with C. *difficile*. Of these, about one in five patients suffered recurrent infection. They found the rate of recurrent C. *difficile* infection was 22.1 percent among people taking medicines to suppress gastric acid. The rate of recurrent C. *difficile* infection was 17.3 percent in people not taking those medicines.

This doesn't mean that you should stop taking medicines to treat heartburn and reflux. In fact, people with coronary artery disease are often prescribed proton pump inhibitors to decrease the risk of bleeding in the stomach and gut, which can be caused by medicines such as aspirin, which is prescribed for the prevention of blood clots. We use one medicine to treat the potential side effects of another—only to find the second medicine has side effects, too.

There are some important caveats of the new study to consider, including the fact that the researchers didn't take into account exactly why patients were using proton pump inhibitors and H2 blockers in the first place. Maybe their reason for taking the medicines, some underlying pathology, could turn out to be the link to recurrent C. *difficile* infection, and the medicine isn't to blame.

The type of study the Mayo Clinic researchers did is called a meta-analysis. It pulls together findings from multiple studies to look for common findings. While powerful in their ability to combine data from thousands of patients across many studies, meta-analyses lump together findings, and the final conclusions sometimes miss important differences in the individual studies.

In this case, the findings show that it might be worth stopping treatment with proton pump inhibitors and H2 blockers in patients already suffering with C. *difficile* or who are at high risk of C. *difficile*. Rates of the infection have skyrocketed over the past decade, and infection with the bacteria is linked to the overuse of antibiotics, which disrupt the balance of good and bad bacteria.

The yearly incidence of recurrent C. *difficile* increased by almost 200 percent from 2001 to 2012, according to a study by researchers at the University of Pennsylvania. Half a million Americans were infected in 2011, according to the Centers for Disease Control and Prevention; 29,000 of them died of C. *difficile* within the first month of their diagnosis.

A Danish study looking at more than 7,000 people recently discharged from the hospital found those taking a proton pump inhibitor were more likely to develop pneumonia. Another study found ICU patients on the medicines were more prone to developing pneumonia. It's thought that by interfering with acid production, proton pump inhibitors compromise the very thing that protects against bacteria. These bacteria are then able to flourish and end up in the body's airways. Another theory is that proton pump inhibitors work by slowing enzymes that reduce the acidity of the esophagus and lungs, making them more prone to infection.

A study published in 2017 found an increased risk of heart failure in patients with coronary artery disease who were taking the medicine to suppress stomach acid. The researchers followed 706 patients with coronary artery disease and who also took medicines such as Prilosec and Nexium. They looked to see which patients had heart attacks, heart failure, and stroke. Patients taking proton pump inhibitors were more likely to suffer heart failure, they found. Proton pump inhibitors suppress stomach acid by blocking the gastric acid pump. But this pump is also present in heart tissue, and studies in rats have found the medicines could affect the way heart muscle contracts.

But there were important caveats in this study, too. Patients who were taking a proton pump inhibitor and found to be more likely to suffer heart failure were also older.

The Mayo Clinic study highlights the fact that there are risks associated with even the seemingly most benign pills. It's always worth evaluating your medicines with your doctor, talking about switching to H2 blockers, if that's right for you, and ditching any unnecessary pills.

20

Were dietary supplements linked to a deadly outbreak of hepatitis?

I n 2013, Sonnette Marras, a 48-year-old mother of seven who lived in Hawaii, decided she wanted to lose weight she had gained during pregnancy. She turned to a weight loss supplement called OxyElite Pro, made by USPLabs and available in health food stores across the United States. A few weeks after she began taking OxyElite, Sonnette became violently ill and was rushed to the hospital, where doctors told her children she had a week left to live. Her liver was shutting down.

Twenty-three more people fell ill with liver swelling in Hawaii after taking the same supplement. As news of the outbreak spread, reports came in from the mainland United States. By the spring of 2014, ninety-seven people in sixteen states were reported sick after taking OxyElite Pro.

Several of them received liver transplants, but when doctors examined Sonnette, they found a tumor in her breast and said she was not eligible for a liver transplant. She died with her family at her bedside.

Every year, 60 percent of Americans use dietary supplements in the hopes of losing weight, gaining muscle, and becoming healthier. And every year, at least 25,000 Americans visit the emergency room because of adverse events linked to these supplements, according to a study published in the *New England Journal of Medicine.*

Dietary supplements are a $30-billion-a-year industry. Not quite medicines, not quite food, dietary supplements fall into a regulatory black hole. One of the most glaring examples of what can go wrong involves USPLabs, which continued to manufacture dietary supplements with an illegal ingredient, one year after that ingredient was deemed unsafe.

The story begins in 1994, when Senators Orrin Hatch and Tom Harkin introduced a federal law, the Dietary Supplement Health and Education Act (DSHEA), which opened the door for supplements to be sold without safety testing.

This means that the pills, powders, and potions on sale across the nation are deemed safe—until someone gets sick. "We don't approve these products for safety or efficacy prior to going to market," says Dr. Daniel Fabricant, director of the Division of Dietary Supplement Programs at the Food and Drug Administration. The FDA regulates foods, medicines, and medical devices, but not dietary supplements.

"They're not like drugs," said Fabricant. "The way the law is, firms don't have to register their products, so dietary supplements come on to the market freely."

It's a huge market. In 2009, 55,000 supplements were on sale in the United States, according to the Government Accountability Office. That's up from 4,000 in 1994, a nearly 1,300 percent increase.

When a supplement is suspected of having caused deaths or illnesses, it's up to the FDA to prove that the supplement is unsafe. "The burden is on us," says Fabricant. "Proving that something caused harm directly is very challenging."

Jacob Geissler has taken full advantage of that challenge with his Dallas sports supplement company. The 37-year-old founded USPLabs in 2006 after graduating with a degree in nutrition from Texas A&M in the mid-1990s.

In between graduating and starting USPLabs, Geissler was indicted in Bexar County in 2003 for possessing thousands of pills containing anabolic steroids. He was ordered to serve ten years of community supervision; he served five of them before his petition for early termination was granted in 2009.

By then, USPLabs was well established. The company became popular for its Jack3d and OxyElite Pro supplements. Both are advertised as simultaneous fat-burners and muscle-builders that will take your workout to the next level. Until July 2013, both contained DMAA, a laboratory-made chemical, which has been illegal in the United States since April 2012.

Company officials said that DMAA is safe. A statement sent to marketers stated that the company was phasing out products containing DMAA "for business reasons."

Originally developed as a nasal decongestant by Eli Lilly in the 1940s, DMAA was removed from the market in 1983 at the company's request. Scientific studies of its effects had demonstrated increases in heart rate and blood pressure, alongside nervousness and tremors. But DMAA enjoyed a comeback after 2006. Touted as a natural derivative of geranium, it became an active ingredient of performance-enhancing and weight loss supplements.

After six deaths and more than 100 reports of sickness were linked to DMAA, it was banned by the FDA in April 2012. But the US Defense Department didn't wait for an FDA ruling. Military officials had banned DMAA four months earlier after the deaths of three soldiers at Fort Bliss, an Army base in Texas. All three soldiers were young, healthy men.

Michael Lee Sparling, one of those soldiers, was a 22-year-old Californian who collapsed after a ten-minute run with his unit in 2011. He had taken the recommended dose of Jack3d, which contains DMAA, before training.

When a fourth soldier died after taking DMAA, the Defense Department convened a safety review panel and conducted a case control study of nearly 2,000 active-duty military personnel. Among the panel's findings: 15.4 percent were taking DMAA; forty soldiers had reported illness to a military doctor after taking the supplement; and two soldiers suffered liver failure. No other cause could be found to explain their illnesses.

There were warning signs in other countries even earlier than the military ban. New Zealand suspended the sale of DMAA in 2008 after it was associated with strokes in four people. DMAA was also banned in Canada, the United Kingdom, and at least six other countries.

In April 2012, four months after the Defense Department's ban, the FDA sent a warning letter to eleven DMAA manufacturers, including USPLabs, stating that DMAA must be removed from all products. Ten companies complied. USPLabs did not. OxyElite Pro and Jack3d continued to be manufactured with DMAA and sold in stores such as GNC.

Even then, it was the Texas Department of State Health Services, not the FDA, that stepped in first. "We embargoed the product at the USPLabs warehouse in Dallas in May [2013] and handed it over to the FDA in June," spokesperson Chris van Deusen said. "Under state law, we can act a little more quickly than the FDA." USPLabs had been illegally making OxyElite Pro and Jack3d with DMAA for thirteen months.

In July, after legal action by the FDA, USPLabs voluntarily destroyed $8.5 million worth of OxyElite Pro and Jack3d at its Dallas facility. But bottles that were already on store shelves stayed there. "We didn't recall product," says the FDA's Fabricant. "But at the same time, in terms of our authority, it was a significant step to get it out of the hands of the distributor and have it voluntarily destroyed."

The largest retailer of dietary supplements, GNC, continued to sell OxyElite Pro and Jack3d until the FDA obtained seizure orders for warehouses in South Carolina and Pennsylvania in June. GNC declined requests for an interview. But in an email to the *New York Times,* a GNC spokesperson said, "It is hard to view this action as anything other than a biased agency action against GNC in retaliation for GNC's stance on DMAA."

Not even the GNC seizures marked the end of OxyElite Pro and Jack3d.

USPLabs, like many dietary supplement manufacturers, presented a moving target. It reformulated OxyElite Pro under the same name without DMAA. This time, it added a new ingredient: aegeline. An extract of the bael tree, which grows in Southeast Asia, aegeline is deemed unsafe by the FDA. The FDA issued a warning on its website: "USPLabs should have informed FDA of its plans to add aegeline to its dietary supplements and it should have established the safety of aegeline in its products. Neither of those things happened."

It was this new formulation of OxyElite Pro that was linked to the fatal outbreak of liver disease that began in Hawaii and spread to the mainland. At least forty-four people were sickened, twenty-two required hospitalization, two needed liver transplants, and one woman—a 48-year-old mother of seven children—died.

The FDA sent a warning letter to USPLabs in October 2013 stating that aegeline was an illegal ingredient. A second warning letter dated November 6 stated that all products containing the illegal ingredient should be recalled. The company voluntarily recalled OxyElite Pro three days later.

GNC again acted consistently. Its stores in Hawaii continued to sell OxyElite Pro, despite a Hawaii Department of Health request to remove the product from shelves. The company later acquiesced.

Dr. Sarah Park worries that there are more undetected cases of liver disease on the mainland. As the state epidemiologist for Hawaii, she was first to be notified of the cluster of liver disease associated with OxyElite Pro. "But we're a small state," she says. "We only have one liver transplant center, and we all talk to each other, so news of these patients got out. We call it the coconut wireless."

Larger states with multiple transplant centers—including Texas, which has fourteen—could miss a similar cluster of patients. Given these problems, it might seem strange that the FDA isn't able to protect Americans. But it's up against a powerful industry that has strong support in Washington.

That takes us back to the 1994 law that allows companies like USPLabs to sell supplements without safety testing, the Dietary Supplement Health and Education Act. Utah's senior senator, Hatch, was the principal author and has been heralded as an ally of the industry ever since. Today, Utah is the Silicon Valley of the dietary supplement industry, providing the state an annual revenue of $7.2 billion.

The second principal author of the law was Iowa's Harkin. His top financial contributor since 1989 is Herbalife International, a dietary supplement company with headquarters in Grand Cayman. Herbalife's political action committee and its employees contributed $87,636 to Harkin's reelection campaign in 2008 and $100,000 to his eponymous public policy institute at Iowa State University in 2011.

Hatch and Harkin's support of the dietary supplement industry has not waned since 1994. In fact, they hit back hard in 2011, when the FDA drafted new guidelines requiring manufacturers to submit a notification for every supplement containing an ingredient that had not been in dietary supplements before 1994. This change would enable the FDA to stay on top of the burgeoning marketplace, rather than only responding to reports of illness and death after the fact.

But in a strongly worded letter to the FDA, Harkin and Hatch complained that this was a "burdensome requirement that would impose substantial, additional costs on manufacturers" and that it "undermined DSHEA." The senators urged the FDA to immediately withdraw the guidance.

Dietary supplements are not getting any safer, scientists say. Liver damage from dietary supplements is on the rise, up from 7 percent of all drug-induced liver illness in 2004 to 20 percent in 2014, according to a study by scientists at the Einstein Medical Center in Philadelphia.

Until the law changes, the burden is on consumers to recognize this sobering fact: Dietary supplements are not tested for safety or efficacy and are considered safe until proven otherwise. A resource-poor, often shackled government agency is doing its best to protect you, but the rules are stacked against it. The dietary supplement market is a place where caveat emptor reigns.

21

Can gay and bisexual men donate blood?

I n 1983, two years into the HIV/AIDS epidemic, the Food and Drug Administration banned gay and bisexual men from ever donating blood in their lifetime. It was a blanket rule that lumped all gay men together as if they are a monolith. It meant a gay man in a monogamous relationship was banned from giving blood, whereas a straight man who had unsafe sex with multiple partners could donate freely.

The rule was designed to prevent transmission of HIV through blood transfusions, the FDA said. Back in the '80s, the agency believed it had good reason to ban men who had sex with men from donating blood: the HIV epidemic was spreading, there was no HIV test and no way of screening blood donations for the virus.

That changed in 1985, when a new test allowed blood donors to be screened for HIV. But it would be another thirty years before the agency's rules caught up, somewhat, with the science. In 2015, the FDA lifted the lifetime ban—but there was a major caveat.

News reports that the ban was completely overturned were exaggerated. It wasn't so much of an overturning as an easing of the restrictions. Gay and bisexual men were now allowed to donate blood but only if they had been celibate for a year. The celibacy rule excludes so many gay men that some activists have said the authorities might as well continue to ban gay men from being blood donors.

If the ban on gay men donating blood were lifted, an additional 360,600 men would likely donate blood each year, according to research by the Williams Institute at the UCLA School of Law. That would amount to an extra 615,300 pints of blood a year.

That blood is needed desperately. Blood shortages occur annually, usually during summer months, when blood drives are less frequent. Demand, on the other hand, does not dwindle. Every two seconds, someone in America needs blood, according to the American Red Cross. A single liver transplant patient can use more than 100 units of blood during surgery.

The FDA's celibacy rule puts the United States in line with Australia, Britain, France, and Sweden, where gay men can donate blood if they have been celibate at least a year. But in Italy, men who have sex with men can donate blood as long as they test negative for HIV and have been practicing safer sex. And in Argentina and Spain, anyone who has had unsafe sex is banned from giving blood, regardless of sexual orientation.

Studies of the Australian blood donation system, when the country switched from a complete ban to a twelve-month deferral, found it was no riskier to use donated blood with the twelve-month deferral in place.

Blood discrimination is as old as blood banking itself.

When Pearl Harbor was bombed in 1941, African Americans lined up to donate blood for those injured in the attacks. They were told to go home. The Red Cross didn't want Black people's blood. Even when it changed its policy the next year and said Black people could donate blood, the Red Cross segregated blood so that white Americans would not receive blood donated by Black Americans.

A Black man was the mastermind behind America's blood transfusion system. Dr. Charles Drew, the "father of the blood bank," was a Black American scientist who set up an experimental blood bank, thought to be one of the first of its kind, at Presbyterian Hospital in New York City in 1939.

Such was Drew's scientific acumen when it came to safely collecting, storing, and delivering blood, that he was flown to the United Kingdom to help the country coordinate transfusions for tens of thousands of soldiers who desperately needed treatment during World War II. Drew was medical director of the US Blood for Britain project, which is said to have saved the lives of tens of thousands of soldiers.

In the United States, Drew established a dried plasma program for the Red Cross in New York and was named assistant director for the Red Cross plasma service. It was the beginning of what would become the National Blood Donor Service, the same service that would refuse to accept Black people's blood.

When the Red Cross stopped segregating blood in 1949, Southern states such as Louisiana and Arkansas continued the practice. Arkansas stopped segregating blood in 1969 and Louisiana in 1972. (Racist blood laws continued though. It wasn't until 1983 that Louisiana overturned a statute that said Blackness was based on a mathematical formula and that anyone with one thirty-second or less "Negro blood" should not be considered Black.)

In South Africa, racial profiling of blood donors occurred after apartheid ended. Blood donated by Black South Africans was thrown away, while blood from white and Indian South Africans was accepted. The blood service said racial profiling was its way of determining which blood donations were most likely to contain HIV, since the virus was much more prevalent among Black South Africans. The blood service's medical director told the South African Press Association that racial profiling of blood donors was the "most logical, medical, ethical and legally defensible system available." But South Africa stopped racially profiling blood donors in 2004 after an international uproar.

The HIV epidemic in the United States disproportionately affects people of color and gay and bisexual men, and the current policy serves to discriminate against queer people, activists say.

In the public health world, we often use the term MSM, or men who have sex with men, instead of gay and bisexual, since it's behavior that determines HIV risk, not a label of gay or bisexual. Interestingly, while the HIV epidemic continues to be focused among the MSM population—in the United States in 2014, MSM accounted for around 2 percent of the population but 70 percent of new infections—there's a difference among MSM blood donors.

According to an FDA report, male donors who report that they are MSM have a lower prevalence of HIV, 0.25 percent, compared to the prevalence of HIV in the general population of MSM, 11–12 percent.

In a 2018 paper, researchers at Columbia University and New York University wrote of the new FDA ruling: "This updated policy is as discriminatory as the lifetime ban and will not significantly increase the number of eligible donors." They called for a shift away from a categorical ban to a system that looked at indicators of risky sex.

On April 2, 2020, as the Covid-19 pandemic swept across the planet, the FDA announced a change in its blood donation guidelines. Because of the greater demand for blood, and "based on recently completed studies and epidemiologic data," the agency said instead of waiting one year after sex with a man, MSM need only wait three months after having sex with a man before donating blood. The same rule applied to women who had been told to wait one year after having sex with a man who had had sex with another man. They also could donate blood after waiting three months.

Medical groups and activists have accused the FDA of demonizing MSM and lumping them in the same group as intravenous drug users. Bans by medical organizations impact the way groups are viewed by the rest of society. In the 1980s, when the FDA banned blood donations from Haitian Americans who had arrived in the United States after 1977, Haitian Americans were scrutinized and stigmatized. After much opposition by human rights organizations and activist groups, the ban was lifted in 1990.

Some argue the current twelve-month celibacy rule is in keeping with rules to protect the blood supply from other infectious diseases including malaria, Zika, and Creutzfeldt-Jakob disease.

For example, anyone who has visited a place with malaria is banned from donating blood for a year; travelers to countries with a Zika epidemic must wait a month before they give blood; and people who lived in the United Kingdom during the mad cow disease crisis are indefinitely banned from donating blood in the United States (that includes me, since I grew up in England).

In the 2015 ruling, the FDA said people with hemophilia and related blood clotting disorders are still banned from donating blood, but not because they pose an increased risk of transmitting HIV, which was the agency's earlier logic.

Now it says the ban exists because hemophiliacs could suffer potential harm from the needles used to take blood.

The FDA said that it made changes to the blood donation policy based on the best available data and that it will "closely monitor the effects" over the next few years. It added that the policy will be reviewed to reflect the most current scientific knowledge. But for now, hundreds of thousands of men in the United States are prohibited from donating blood, and many scientists believe the FDA's rules are not in line with scientific evidence.

Diseases such as HIV don't discriminate based on a person's ethnicity, race, or sexual orientation. It's not about who you are, it's what you do that puts you at risk for HIV. The FDA and other blood organizations should adopt risk-based blood donation policies instead of discriminating against broad groups of people.

22

Are e-cigarettes helpful or harmful?

I n the spring of 2019, young people, mostly young men in Illinois and Wisconsin, began to fall sick with a strange lung disease. They coughed, struggled to catch their breath, and some ended up on ventilators inside intensive care units. By August, a young man died of the lung disease in Illinois. Another died from the same condition in Oregon. A boy died in New York in October, becoming the first teenager to die from the mysterious disease.

Public health experts interviewed the cluster of sick men and the families of those who had died and discovered they had something in common: they smoked e-cigarettes. By November 2019, 2,290 people had fallen sick with the lung disease, and nearly fifty people had died across twenty-five states and the District of Columbia. The Centers for Disease Control and Prevention labeled the condition EVALI, or e-cigarette or vaping product use–associated lung injury.

Investigators seeking clues found that ingredients in the liquids that were being smoked in e-cigarettes could be the culprit. But this discovery sparked a massive debate. Around the world, medical experts have been in disagreement over the safety of e-cigarettes. Some doctors hail them as the best tool to help smokers give up cigarettes, while some health agencies have declared e-cigarettes responsible for creating a new generation of nicotine addicts. England's leading public health agency, Public Health England, recommends that doctors should be allowed to prescribe e-cigarettes for smoking cessation. Some British politicians have called for e-cigarette laws to be relaxed.

The World Health Organization has argued that too little is known about the long-term effects of using e-cigarettes, that the nicotine in them is addictive, and that some flavorings in e-cigarettes can cause irritation and inflammation of the airways. In 2019, San Francisco became the first US city to ban the sale of e-cigarettes, with city officials declaring an "abdication of responsibility" by the Food and Drug Administration in regulating the products. In September of 2019, as the outbreak of EVALI continued to grow, the FDA conducted its own investigation and found vitamin E acetate in the cannabis vaping products of nearly every person sick with EVALI in New York. Vitamin E is safe to ingest or apply to the skin and is found in food and lotions, but it is not safe to inhale. The FDA said it was being added as a thickening agent and to possibly increase levels of THC, the main psychogenic compound in cannabis. Two months after the FDA's discovery, the CDC announced a breakthrough. It found vitamin E acetate in the lungs of twenty-nine people with EVALI.

Electronic cigarettes, or e-cigarettes, also known as vaporizers and vape pens, are battery-powered smoking devices that contain a vaporizer, which heats up the liquid in a cartridge. That liquid usually contains nicotine, flavorings, and other additives. The heating element in most e-cigarettes is activated by inhaling, while others have a manual switch.

There are two main types of e-cigarettes, open system or open tanks and closed system or closed tanks. In an open tank, the liquid that is vaporized can be manually refilled, and there's usually a removable mouthpiece. In a closed tank e-cigarette, ready-made refills are screwed directly onto the battery. Open tank e-cigarettes are the most popular type of e-cigarette.

In the United States, the FDA says there's an "epidemic" of vaping among teenagers and e-cigarette manufacturers aren't doing enough to combat underage use of their products. Some public health experts in the United States have called e-cigarettes an emerging public health threat, quickly undoing decades of antismoking campaigning.

Why can't everyone agree? For one, e-cigarettes have only been around since 2003, when the first commercially successful e-cigarette was created by Hon Lik, a Chinese pharmacist and smoker. It's said that Lik invented the electronic cigarette after his father—a heavy smoker, like Lik—died from lung cancer. Lik may have been inspired by Herbert Gilbert, who patented a "smokeless, non-tobacco cigarette" four decades earlier in 1965.

While the number of cigarette consumers is steadily decreasing—down from 1.14 billion in 2000 to 1.1 billion people globally, according to market research group, Euromonitor—the use of e-cigarettes is rising dramatically.

The number of e-cigarette smokers has increased fivefold in a five-year period, going up from 7 million in 2011 to 35 million in 2016, according to Euromonitor. The company predicts that 55 million people will be smoking e-cigarettes by 2021.

The industry was worth an estimated $22.6 billion globally in 2018, compared to $4.2 billion in 2013, with the United Kingdom, Japan, and the United States establishing themselves as the biggest markets for vaping products. In these three countries, e-cigarette users spent more than $16 billion on vaping products in 2016.

E-cigarettes have overtaken regular cigarettes to become the most popular tobacco product for American teenagers. One in five 18- to 24-year-olds in the United States has used an e-cigarette, according to the CDC.

Cigarettes contain thousands of compounds, at least seventy of which are known carcinogens. They also contain carbon monoxide, arsenic, and other poisons. E-cigarettes, on the other hand, contain far fewer compounds overall, perhaps hundreds of chemicals instead of the thousands found in cigarettes.

The main ingredients of vaping fluid are glycerol and propylene glycol, which many say are harmless when inhaled. But employees of theaters and movie sets who use these chemicals to create mist and fog special effects, have reported breathing problems, perhaps linked to long-term exposure of propylene glycol.

In studies, some e-cigarette vapor has been found to contain very low levels of nitrosamines, which have been linked to cancer. Other studies have shown that the vapor contains toxic chemicals, including acetaldehyde and formaldehyde, and some flavorings, especially cinnamon, butter, and vanilla, contain free radicals, which can damage DNA.

The relative novelty of e-cigarettes means a lack of long-term safety data. For this reason, some scientists have called out politicians and public health agencies advocating for the expanded use of e-cigarettes.

In a 2018 report, Public Health England said it was plausible that e-cigarettes were responsible for the highest ever rate of people who had successfully given up smoking cigarettes in England. But there's conflicting evidence about the effectiveness of e-cigarettes as a tool for smoking cessation.

In the same report, Public Health England goes on to say that of seven meta-analyses of smoking cessation, two found a positive effect of e-cigarettes on quitting smoking, four were inconclusive, and one found a negative effect. In a 2018 study of more than 6,000 smokers, researchers at the University of Pennsylvania found e-cigarettes were not useful in helping cigarette smokers kick the habit. (Cash incentives were.)

There's a widespread belief among e-cigarette users that vaping is safe and can help with quitting regular cigarettes. In a 2016 report by Ernst & Young, with Nicoventures, a start-up of British American Tobacco, research conducted in seven European and Asian countries showed the most common reason for smoking e-cigarettes was that they were considered "less harmful than regular cigarettes." Almost half of all regular users said they were using e-cigarettes to give up smoking cigarettes.

But in the United States, where e-cigarette use has increased 900 percent since 2011 among high schoolers and where nearly 6 percent of middle school students say they have smoked an e-cigarette in the last year, public health officials say vaping is introducing more young people to the idea of smoking and could lead to cigarette use.

In a 2016 report, US Surgeon General Dr. Vivek Murthy, said young people are at highest risk of becoming addicted to the nicotine in e-cigarettes. Nicotine impacts brain development, which continues until people are in their midtwenties.

Nicotine can affect the prefrontal cortex, a part of the brain that is the last to mature. Studies have shown that exposure to nicotine during the teenage years increases a person's risk of developing psychiatric illnesses and attention deficit disorders.

Some scientists are worried that teens who smoke e-cigarettes are more likely to go on to smoke regular cigarettes. Scientists at the University of Hawaii found e-cigarettes promoted cigarette smoking among young people. The researchers interviewed more than 2,000 high school students in 2013 and again a year later. About a third of those students said they had tried an e-cigarette by the time they were first interviewed. A year later, students who had previously smoked e-cigarettes were about three times more likely to have tried a regular cigarette, compared with those who had not used e-cigarettes.

In Britain, the Royal College of Physicians (RCP) says smokers should be given e-cigarettes to help them give up smoking regular cigarettes. In a report published in 2016, the United Kingdom's leading medical body said e-cigarettes are not a gateway to smoking and should be used as a smoking cessation aid.

In 2014, a study in Britain found that those who used e-cigarettes were 60 percent more likely to be successful in giving up cigarettes than those who went cold turkey or used nicotine patches and gum. But some experts say it's too soon to tell if e-cigarettes help people quit smoking, although the evidence so far has swayed the RCP and Public Health England. E-cigarettes have now outpaced nicotine gum and patches to become the most popular tool for smoking cessation in Britain.

The FDA has not licensed e-cigarettes as a tool for smoking cessation. In fact, the agency offers a warning about the risks posed by e-cigarettes. In 2009, the FDA analyzed the liquid contents in two leading brands of e-cigarettes. It found them to contain chemicals that can cause cancer, including nitrosamines, and a toxic chemical found in antifreeze.

In 2018, the FDA found prescription medications inside vaping fluid. Erectile dysfunction drugs, Viagra and Cialis, which should be available only with a prescription, were discovered inside e-cigarette liquids made by the Chinese e-cigarette maker, HelloCig Electronic Technology. The medicines could dangerously lower blood pressure, the agency said.

There's also a threat of injury when the battery inside an e-cigarette overheats. More than two dozen people were injured by exploding e-cigarettes from 2009 to 2014, according to the US Fire Administration. Doctors say those injured suffer flame burns, chemical burns, and blast injuries.

Public health experts continue to disagree about the safety of e-cigarettes, leaving the more than 35 million people who use them in the middle of a heated debate. They may be healthier than smoking cigarettes, but that doesn't mean they are harmless.

By February 2020, the outbreak of EVALI had spread to every state in the United States, and the CDC said it would officially count only those people who were sick enough to be hospitalized with EVALI or die from the disease. By that count, the CDC reported nearly 3,000 people who had been hospitalized and sixty-eight deaths. But federal authorities have been slow to regulate the products; in fact it was only in 2016 that the FDA was given regulatory powers over e-cigarettes. In the absence of federal leadership, the United States has a patchwork of vaping regulations that vary massively by state, leaving individual consumers to figure out what is safe and what is not.

23

Is marijuana a performance-enhancing drug for athletes?

I f you're picturing yourself in college taking bong hits, sinking into the sofa, and missing deadlines, you're probably wondering why highly competitive pro athletes would use cannabis. Times have changed.

Alongside protein powders and workout supplements, some athletes and their trainers are smoking, eating, and anointing themselves with cannabis oils, tinctures, and edibles. And nowadays, weed connoisseurs discuss cannabis strains the way sommeliers compare grape varieties.

The key components of cannabis are tetrahydrocannabinol (THC), which gives the feeling of being high, and cannabinol (CBN) and cannabidiol (CBD), which are not known for being psychoactive but are likely to have anti-inflammatory effects that could help alleviate pain and nausea.

I say likely because there's not a lot of scientific data about cannabis, and this makes our question—is cannabis a performance-enhancing drug?—difficult to answer.

Data are limited because cannabis is illegal in much of the world. In the United States it's a schedule 1 drug, so although at the time I'm writing this in

2018 it's legal to use cannabis recreationally in nine states and Washington, DC, and legal to use medical marijuana in thirty states; it's still hard for scientists to get cannabis into the lab to study. The Drug Enforcement Administration considers cannabis to have "no currently accepted medical use." It groups cannabis with heroin and LSD.

What we do know is some athletes use cannabis, and they say it helps relieve anxiety and facilitates focus. Let's start back in 1998, when Canadian snowboarder Ross Rebagliati nearly lost his Olympic medal after testing positive for cannabis. He appealed and won back his medal because, at the time, cannabis was not on the banned-substance list.

It was added to the list a year later, not because it was known to give athletes an unfair advantage, but because it was illegal in much of the world. Rebagliati is from Canada, which was one of the first nations to allow medical marijuana use, in 2001. He's taking advantage of that ruling and has set up shop as a dispenser of medical marijuana.

"For me, whether you are skiing, or snowboarding, or riding a road bike, or working out at the gym, [marijuana] puts you in the moment. You get in a zone where you can give it 110 percent," he says on his website.

Cannabis is banned by the World Anti-Doping Agency, which oversees drug testing for the Olympics. It's also banned by the US Anti-Doping Agency and the National Collegiate Athletic Association.

But the World Anti-Doping Agency recently changed the rules regarding how much cannabis was allowed in an athlete's blood. The threshold was raised from 15 ng/ml to 150 ng/ml, which gives an indication that the agency is concerned about athletes smoking during the games but not in the weeks prior to the competition.

Back when Rebagliati first lost his Olympic medal, his blood concentration of cannabis was 17.8 ng/ml. He said the result was from secondhand smoke, a statement he stands by today. He was quick to defend Olympic champion Michael Phelps in 2009 when a photo of a 23-year-old Phelps taking a bong hit went viral. Phelps isn't the only Olympic athlete who has admitted to a history of cannabis use. Some have even been banned for using it. In 2012, American judoka Nicholas Delpopolo was banned from competing in the London Olympics after testing positive for cannabis.

Because it's a schedule 1 drug, there aren't many well-designed studies looking at the effect of cannabis on humans. Much of the research comes from experiments in rodents, but there are differences between cannabinoid receptors in mice and men.

Some evidence comes from people who admit to self-medicating with cannabis, even in places where it's illegal. That's one way we know that cannabis can be effective in the treatment of multiple sclerosis. A study of 112 MS patients in the United States and United Kingdom in the 1990s found cannabis improved symptoms of pain, depression, and tremors in more than 90 percent of them.

It's been reported that cannabis can alleviate anxiety, cause euphoria, and improve sociability, which could help with the stress of playing competitive sports. But it can also cause paranoia, a rapid heartbeat, disrupt hand-eye coordination, and decrease reaction time—not what you need during a high-stakes game.

Still, while some athletes I have spoken to report taking cannabis before a game, citing its ability to help with focus and pain tolerance, others say they would never dream of playing while high. Instead, some have told me they smoke, vape, or eat cannabis to help facilitate a good night's sleep before a game.

It's possible to use cannabis without getting high. Preparations that limit the amount of THC while delivering a hit of CBD claim to alleviate nausea, reduce anxiety, and help with mood and sleep.

If you live in a state where it's legal, cannabis is now available in energy bars and edibles as well as in formulations for smoking and vaping. You can rub cannabis-infused balms and ointments into fatigued muscles to aid relaxation and pain relief.

In an effort to destigmatize cannabis use and demonstrate that weed users are athletes, too, Jim McAlpine started the 420 Games, a series of five-mile runs in California, Colorado, Oregon, and Washington.

Some pro athletes are putting their careers on the line by advocating for cannabis as a pain management option. As the United States battles a deadly and devastating epidemic of deaths from prescription painkillers, former Baltimore Ravens player Eugene Monroe publicly asked the National Football League to let players use medical marijuana.

The Ravens issued a statement saying they did not stand behind Monroe's request and in June 2016, they released him from the team. It's unclear whether Monroe was let go because of injuries or because of his stance on medical marijuana.

It's interesting to note that the drugs responsible for killing tens of thousands of Americans each year, drugs like Vicodin and Oxycontin, are legal and sit in a lower, less prohibitive DEA category than cannabis. While cannabis remains a schedule 1 drug in the United States, getting any meaningful data on its effects on athletic performance and overall health may be nearly impossible.

Canada may prove to be the antidote to that problem. In the months leading up to the legalization of cannabis in Canada in October 2018, funding for cannabis research began to increase. In July 2018, the Canadian Institutes of Health Research, Canada's federal funding agency for health research, announced CA$3 million for cannabis research.

Canadian scientists say legalization could allow them to address the gaps in our understanding of how cannabis affects the brain and body. M-J Milloy, a research scientist in the Centre on Substance Use at the University of British Columbia, told reporters: "What we, as scientists, have not been able to do is try to figure out what those risks and benefits are in an open way."

Milloy added: "The hope is that legalization of cannabis will take the shackles off scientific inquiry and will allow us to ask and answer the sort of questions we should have been asking twenty, thirty, forty years ago." That could include a deeper understanding of the drug's impact on athletic performance.

24

Did a morning sickness pill for pregnant women cause birth defects in thousands of babies?

I n the late 1950s, pregnant women in the United Kingdom, Mexico, Japan, Germany, Canada, and dozens more countries were offered a pill for morning sickness. The pill wasn't new, it was thalidomide, a medicine already popular for soothing fraught nerves, headaches, and insomnia, but for the first time thalidomide was being marketed as a cure for morning sickness.

Lauded for its safety—scientists said it was impossible to overdose on it—the drug was even available over the counter in many countries. Pleased to have a new treatment for morning sickness, some women swallowed thalidomide once or twice during pregnancy, others took it every day for weeks.

Months later, tens of thousands of babies were born with shrunken arms and legs, missing fingers, and other severe birth defects, known as phocomelia. In one of the greatest tragedies in the history of the pharmaceutical industry, thalidomide caused severe birth defects in babies and may have caused the deaths of thousands of fetuses.

Growing up in England in the 1980s, I would see thalidomide survivors shopping for groceries or lining up for tickets at the cinema, and being a curious child, I would ask my mum who they were and why their arms and legs looked different from mine.

Rosie Moriarty Simmonds is one of those survivors. Rosie was born in the United Kingdom in 1960 to a mother who was prescribed thalidomide. Rosie said her mother, Mena, suffered from asthma and morning sickness and her doctor said thalidomide would alleviate her nausea and vomiting. Rosie is a writer, broadcaster, and disability campaigner who tells her story to raise awareness about the thousands affected by thalidomide.

"I was born on a Sunday at about 10:00 at night, delivered by a student doctor and clearly when I was delivered there was a hushed silence and shock in the theater," Rosie said. "And then I was taken away straightaway and my mum was almost immediately sedated. She assumed I'd been born stillborn."

Rosie thinks her mother was sedated because the doctors thought she wouldn't be able to cope with the shock of seeing her baby. "I've got two fingers that literally come out of each shoulder and although they're not that long, they are useful. And I use my mouth a lot and my teeth a lot," says Rosie. In total she has four fingers and thirteen toes. "I'm a disabled woman who is missing arms and legs caused by the drug thalidomide."

A few days after Rosie was born, her mother, roused from the sedation, pulled the drip out of her arm and crawled toward her baby. "I was wrapped up head to toe," Rosie said. "They had just prior to that tried to explain I had been born with little arms and legs and when she started to slowly look under the blankets, she looked at me, looked at my face and said, 'Well, isn't she beautiful. She's all mine.'"

But many babies weren't welcomed with that kind of acceptance. Rosie says half of all babies born with defects because of thalidomide in the United Kingdom were abandoned or adopted in the United Kingdom. Rosie's parents were told by priests and hospital workers that they should leave their baby and start all over again.

They didn't listen. Instead her parents started on a years-long course of treatments to try and help Rosie overcome her disabilities. Using prosthetics and physical therapy, doctors tried to get a young Rosie to walk. "My right leg is actually more like a shin bone than a thigh bone so it's not even connected properly through like a ball and socket hip, so throwing one leg and dragging the other, so it wasn't pretty." Metal prosthetics were attached to her bones. "It was very much like walking on stilts without a net beneath you and without arms to be able to balance. I spent more time on my face or backside than I did upright and trying to walk. Not easy."

The world the thalidomide babies grew up in was not kind to children with disabilities. "When I was a baby my mum got me out to go to a shop and I'm wrapped up in the pram and a lady came along and quite often like they do looked in and said 'what a lovely baby' and for some reason pulled the blanket back a little bit and when she saw I just had two little fingers went screaming up the road singing 'it's a freak.'"

A MEDICAL TRAGEDY

Thalidomide was first made by the German drug company, Chemie Grünenthal, in 1954. Four years later, the medicine arrived in the United Kingdom under the brand name Distaval. In the more than forty countries in which it was sold, it was labeled Distaval Forte, Contergan, Tensival, Valgraine, and other names.

Chemie Grünenthal marketed its over-the-counter medicine as safe for everyone, "even during pregnancy." It said it "could not find a dose high enough to kill a rat."

Two years later, in 1956, a worker at Chemie Grünenthal had a baby born with severe birth defects. The father of the child had been given samples of thalidomide for his pregnant wife. But no one made a link between the medicine and the baby's disabilities.

That connection was made by an Australian doctor in May 1961. Dr. William McBride, an obstetrician at a Sydney hospital, delivered a baby with birth defects, including malformed arms. In the coming weeks, he delivered two more babies with similar defects. In December, he wrote a letter to the medical journal the *Lancet,* making the connection that all of the babies' mothers had taken thalidomide, a drug he had prescribed. The doctor ended the letter with a question: "Have any of your readers seen similar abnormalities in babies delivered of women who have taken this drug during pregnancy?"

In November 1961 in Germany, Dr. Widukind Lenz, made the same discovery. Lenz found babies all over the country had been born with defects to mothers who had taken thalidomide. A German newspaper reported that 161 babies had been born with thalidomide-related birth defects and that some adults taking the medicine had suffered a type of nerve damage called peripheral neuritis.

Chemie Grünenthal ignored the earlier warnings. Reluctantly, it pulled the drug from shelves in November 1961. The next month, the British distributor did the same. By March 1962, thalidomide was either banned or withdrawn from most countries in which it had been available. Doctors noted a dramatic decrease in the number of babies born with phocomelia in the year after thalidomide was withdrawn.

By then, thousands of babies had suffered birth defects. The exact number may never be known. "There is no absolute figure for how many babies were affected by thalidomide as many were miscarried, still born or died soon after birth," says the Thalidomide Society, a British organization that supports families affected by the tragedy. It says more than 24,000 babies were affected by thalidomide globally, 2,000 of whom were in the United Kingdom. An estimated 6,000 babies were affected in Germany, where 2,000 were said to have survived.

The Thalidomide Society cites experts who "conservatively estimate that those babies still-born and miscarried, due to thalidomide, would add a further 123,000 worldwide of which 10,000 would have been in the UK. These figures do not include those babies born alive who became victims of state infanticide and so were never registered."

Because thalidomide also appeared in children's cough medicines—sometimes as an unlabeled ingredient—it stayed in homes and on shelves long after it was banned or pulled from the market. In the United Kingdom, at least twenty children were born late in 1962 with thalidomide-related birth defects, many months after the drug had been withdrawn.

How does a drug meant to cure morning sickness cause birth defects? The answer is in the chemistry.

Some molecules exist in two forms, where each is a mirror image of the other. It's a phenomenon known as chirality and it's kind of like our right and left hands, which are similar in shape but are not superimposable, something you can demonstrate by trying to put your right hand in your left glove and vice versa.

Thalidomide is a chiral molecule, meaning it comes in both a right-handed and a left-handed configuration. The right-handed version of the molecule works as a sedative and morning sickness treatment. The left-handed version causes birth defects if taken in the first few months of pregnancy. The problem can't be solved by giving people only the right-handed version because inside the body the right-handed version of thalidomide is converted into the left-handed version.

The left-handed version causes a type of birth defect known as phocomelia, where the long bones of the limbs are short or misshapen. Some babies born to mothers who took thalidomide had fused fingers and fewer than ten fingers. Their legs were clubbed or turned inward with extra toes. Many of the babies had cleft palates or missing ears, and internal organs including the heart and genitals, were also affected.

In 2010, Japanese researchers at the Tokyo Institute of Technology discovered exactly how the left-handed version of thalidomide causes birth defects. The team gave thalidomide to zebrafish and chick embryos and found that development of the zebrafish fins, equivalent to human arms, and the chicks' hearing apparatus, equivalent to human ears, were severely stunted. The scientists discovered that thalidomide binds to a protein called cereblon and inhibits growth factors and enzymes needed for limb development.

Now aged from their midfifties to early sixties, an estimated 3,000 to 6,000 survivors of one of the biggest medical scandals in history are alive today, including nearly 500 living in the United Kingdom, around 300 in Japan, and nearly 50 in Australia.

But a very different situation unfolded in the United States, where there are likely zero people affected by the thalidomide scandal. It's all thanks to one woman who saved millions of babies from the harmful effects of the drug.

A DIFFERENT STORY IN AMERICA

My American friends didn't grow up noticing thalidomide survivors shopping for groceries or asking their parents to explain why their limbs were shaped differently. That's all because of one woman.

On Monday August 1, 1960, Dr. Frances Oldham Kelsey, known as Frankie, started a new job at the Food and Drug Administration just outside of

Washington, DC. Frankie was 46 years old, a medical doctor trained in Canada, and had moved to the United States because she couldn't find work in Canada.

A month into her new job, a file was dropped on Frankie's desk. It was an application to approve a new medicine, thalidomide, manufactured in the United States by a company called Merrell.

The system back then dictated that Frankie had sixty days to say yes or no to the drug. If she became busy and missed the sixty-day deadline, the drug would automatically be approved.

Frankie figured the application for this new medicine had been given to her, a woman and a new employee, because it seemed so cut and dried. A pill already used in much of the world as a sedative—what could go wrong with that?

But looking through the file, Frankie was unconvinced and unimpressed. The FDA at the time didn't require drug companies to submit clinical trial data, and Merrell had submitted information that Frankie deemed anecdotal and unscientific.

She asked Merrell for more evidence of the drug's safety, not just quotes from doctors who felt thalidomide was safe. Merrell was not happy. Executives there pressured Frankie to approve thalidomide because Christmas was fast approaching and they wanted their drug on shelves in time for the season, when sedatives and sleeping pills sold well in America.

The drug's maker pointed to thalidomide's success in Europe. But Frankie pushed for more data. "I held my ground. I just wouldn't approve it," she said to reporters, years later.

Then, six months later, sitting in her office at the FDA, Frankie was looking through the pages of the *British Medical Journal* when she spotted a letter by a British doctor. The doctor described adult patients who had taken thalidomide and developed a painful nerve disease called peripheral neuritis.

The reports of nerve damage got Frankie wondering: If thalidomide could damage an adult's nerves, what might it do to a developing fetus? She pushed back at Merrell, asking the drug company for more data on thalidomide's safety, especially since it was saying the drug was safe for pregnant women.

For a year, Frankie refused to give in to their pressure. By then, doctors such as McBride in Australia and Lenz in Germany, were discovering the harm thalidomide could do to an unborn baby. By the time the drug was pulled from shelves around the world, Frankie still had not approved the application Merrell was insisting she sign.

Had the drug's application landed on someone else's desk, had Frankie bowed to the drug maker's pressure, thalidomide could have been taken by millions of pregnant women across the United States. Instead, seventeen babies were born with thalidomide-related disabilities in the country, each of them to mothers who were offered samples of the unapproved drug by their doctors. In Frankie's native Canada, more than a hundred babies were born with thalidomide-related birth defects.

Frankie's thoroughness, her unwillingness to be bullied or hurried, not only saved the lives of countless babies but also reshaped the way the FDA approved medicines. Soon after the thalidomide scandal unfolded, the agency instituted new rules that meant drug companies had to provide clinical trial data on the safety and efficacy of their medicines.

Thalidomide survivors are in their fifties now. For thousands of them, receiving compensation for the harm they suffered in one of the biggest medical tragedies in history is proving to be a lifelong struggle. The Canadian government pays between CA\$25,000 to CA\$100,000 to 120 surviving thalidomide survivors. Some of the more than 400 British survivors of the thalidomide tragedy also receive compensation from the government. Others have received compensation from the drug maker or distributors.

In Spain, a court ruled that Chemie Grünenthal should pay around 40 million euros to a few dozen survivors. That decision was later overturned when the court said the statute of limitations for the case had expired. For some survivors, it's hard to prove that their mothers took the medicine during pregnancy. Grünenthal said it "deeply regrets the impact of thalidomide on all those affected, their mothers, and their families and friends."

Rosie says it seems as if no one has been held accountable for what happened to her and tens of thousands of pregnant women and their babies. "Neither the government or the drug companies have accepted responsibility or liability for the damage they did to thalidomide people—and their families—because the damage extends beyond us, it's our parents, it's to the parents who kept their children and didn't. Our siblings, and then there's thousands of babies that didn't survive."

A NEW GENERATION OF THALIDOMIDE BABIES

You might expect Rosie's generation to be the last to live with the legacy of the thalidomide scandal, but thalidomide's story is not over. The drug is still used in countries, including Mexico and Brazil, where it was relicensed in 1965 years after it was banned or pulled from the market in dozens of other countries.

In Brazil, thalidomide is used to treat skin lesions caused by the bacterial infection leprosy. Nearly 6 million thalidomide pills were given to people across the country during 2005 to 2010, to treat the 30,000 new cases of leprosy diagnosed each year.

Despite its history of birth defects, Brazilian women have been taking it while pregnant. At least 100 babies have been born with disabilities caused by the drug, according to researchers at Universidade Federal do Rio Grande do Sul who looked at the birth records of 17.5 million babies born in Brazil during 2005 to 2010.

Advocates for the medicine argue that it is the best treatment for leprosy and that thalidomide's benefits outweigh its risks. Brazilian regulations require bottles of thalidomide to be marked as dangerous during pregnancy, and women can only be prescribed the drug if they are using two forms of birth control.

Thalidomide is also being used in the United States. In 1991, scientists at Rockefeller University in New York discovered thalidomide inhibits a protein called tumor necrosis factor alpha. Gilla Kaplan, Jane Tramontana, and others at Rockefeller University published papers in the 1990s stating thalidomide "is emerging as a useful agent in the management of several complications of disease due to human immunodeficiency virus (HIV)." Those complications included painful oral ulcers as well as wasting of the muscles. There were also papers showing the drug could help patients with tuberculosis and Crohn's disease.

A biotech company called Celgene in New Jersey began to make thalidomide and branded the drug, Thalomid. In 2006 it was approved for the treatment of multiple myeloma, a cancer of a type of blood cells called plasma cells in the bone marrow. Combined with a steroid to create a drug called Revlimid, it's now the preferred treatment for multiple myeloma, despite its cost of more than $163,000 a year.

While it's dangerous for developing fetuses, it seems thalidomide is also bad news for the blood vessels that feed cancer cells. Tumors are notorious for forging their own blood supplies, and thalidomide stops the formation of new blood vessels that would otherwise nourish the cancer cells. In fact, thalidomide's ability to block those new blood vessels could help explain another way it stunts limb growth in a fetus.

Doctors hope that understanding exactly how thalidomide harms a growing baby could help make a form of the drug that is still useful for the treatment of leprosy and cancer—but safe.

25

Is there lead in your lipstick?

I n 2010, the Food and Drug Administration, which oversees some aspects of cosmetic safety, asked Frontier Global Sciences, Inc. to test 400 lipsticks for lead contamination. From drugstore brands to high-end cosmetics companies, lead was found in hundreds of lipsticks. Some L'Oreal lipsticks contained the heavy metal, as did designer brands such as NARS, whose lipsticks sell for up to $32. Even a lip shimmer sold by Burt's Bees, a brand that touts itself as "natural," was found to contain lead at nearly three parts per million.

Lead is a naturally occurring metal in the earth's crust, but unlike metals such as iron, zinc, and copper, which are critical to human health, even small amounts of lead are toxic. Children are most vulnerable to lead poisoning because their bodies absorb more of the metal. In children, lead can cause a lower IQ, behavioral issues including criminal behaviors that continue into adulthood, stunted growth, deafness, seizures, and death.

Because lead is found in the environment, the FDA says it can't be helped that it turns up in cosmetics. To the agency, small amounts of lead are considered acceptable in cosmetics. It regulates the safety of dyes used in makeup. Besides dyes, other ingredients and additives contained in makeup do not need FDA approval.

Typically, the agency permits the use of dyes that contain lead at concentrations of ten to twenty parts per million. But after its review, it asked manufacturers of lipsticks with high levels of lead to take their products off the shelves. In 2016, the FDA issued guidance recommending that lipsticks and other cosmetics should contain no more than ten parts per million of lead.

Lead can be absorbed through the skin or licked off the lips. Once inside the body, lead stays in the blood for only a matter of months before it is absorbed by the bones. It can hang around in the bones for years, even decades. That makes it hard to test for lead in the blood. But when a woman is pregnant, lead is released from bones and it crosses the placenta to poison the unborn baby. Pregnant women exposed to lead can give birth prematurely and have babies that are smaller than usual.

Before we knew it was toxic, lead was added to cosmetics to give the skin a bright glow. Queen Elizabeth I used a powder called ceruse, a mix of vinegar and lead, to hide her smallpox scars. A similar powder was found in ancient China as early as 1600 BC.

Cleopatra and ancient Egyptians used kohl to draw dramatic lines around their eyes. The kohl was packed with lead salts. Women living in the Roman Empire and sixteenth-century English women powdered their faces with cosmetics full of lead dust. It might have been beautifying in the short term, but in the long run, lead caused their teeth to turn black and hair to fall out.

What we now recognize as lipstick came to be in the late 1800s in France. That's when sticks of pigmented waxes were sold wrapped in silk paper. Those early versions of lipstick contained fat from deer and were colored with a pigment made from carmine dye, which contained crushed insects. Those dead bugs are still used to make some lipsticks. You might find carmine in bright red ones.

Nowadays lead is not the only contaminant hiding in lipstick. In a study published in 2013, researchers discovered aluminum, chromium, manganese, and cadmium lurking in cosmetics. They found that women who apply contaminated lipsticks and lip glosses two to three times per day ingest more than a safe amount of these metals. And that's not taking into account those of us who reapply lipstick more often.

People who wear lipstick consume 24 milligrams of it every day. If you reapply a few times a day, you consume 87 milligrams, according to a study by researchers at the University of California, Berkeley.

Cadmium, one of the contaminants that's been found in some cosmetics, is used in batteries. It can cause chills, fevers, and general flu-like symptoms and is known to cause cancer. It's not purposefully added to lipstick, but like chromium, it can end up there because the dyes and machines used to make cosmetics sometimes contain these metals.

It's not just lipsticks that contain toxins. Some eyeliners are so densely packed with lead that the metal makes up half the weight of the eyeliner. A case of lead poisoning in a child in Boston in 2011 happened because an eyeliner containing more than 80 percent lead was used on the child. Be wary of eyeliners such as kohl, kajal, surma, and tiro.

Lead is also used in some hair dyes called progressive hair colors. These hair dyes are used over time to cover gray and give what some consider a more natural appearance. Unlike other lead-containing cosmetics, progressive hair dyes must include a warning message on the box.

So are you poisoning yourself with lead and a long list of toxic metals every time you lick your ruby lips? You can check out the list of 400 lipsticks tested by the FDA and its partners for more information on lead contamination. Be aware that many brands are missing from that list because they were not included in the analysis.

The Campaign for Safe Cosmetics, which lobbies for less-toxic makeup, offers advice on its website on which ingredients to avoid when shopping for lipstick, shampoo, conditioner, and other products.

Besides the potential risk of lead exposure from lipsticks, there have been Instagram trends of melting kids' crayons with coconut oil to make vibrant lipsticks and eyeliners at home. In 2016 the trend was touted as the hot new thing but was actually a rehashed trend that had been around for a while. The idea is simple: melt a scoop of coconut oil in a pan, add a crayon of your choosing, and stir. After all, even the fanciest lipsticks are simply paraffin wax and pigments.

But is it safe to paint your face with melted children's crayons?

In light of the Instagram videos, brands such as Crayola issued warnings. "Although our products are nontoxic, we do not recommend using them to make eyeliner, lipstick or other makeup and strongly discourage their use in this manner . . . They are not designed, tested or approved for this use." Then it capitalized on the trend. In 2018, Crayola launched its own makeup line featuring dozens of face and lip crayons. The products were sold in the brand's iconic crayon box packaging.

Cosmetics today are safer than they have ever been, and there's no need to ditch makeup altogether. Check out the FDA's list of cosmetics included in its study of lead contamination to see which lipsticks have the lowest levels.

Should you feel the urge to color your face with crayons, it's best to stick to the ones that are manufactured as cosmetics. While many crayons are marketed as nontoxic, they are intended for use on paper, not skin.

26

Why do immigrants in America live longer than American-born people?

Hispanic immigrants living in the United States have higher rates of poverty, lower rates of education, and are less likely to have health insurance compared to people born in the United States. But despite those odds, immigrants live at least two and a half years longer than white people born in the United States and, in some states, nearly eight years longer than US-born African Americans.

This longevity phenomenon is called the Hispanic paradox, and understanding it could help everyone live a longer life. The term was coined in 1986 by Dr. Kyriakos Markides, professor of aging studies at the University of Texas Medical Branch in Galveston, when he was studying the health of Mexicans in the Southwest. "It's been many years since we discovered this, and people still haven't figured it out," he says.

Back in the '80s, Markides's research showed that the health of Hispanics in the Southwest resembled that of white Americans, although Hispanics were poorer, more likely to be unemployed, and had less access to health care. "It was so paradoxical," he says. "Here's a group that has a similar socioeconomic status to African-Americans but their health resembles the health of non-Hispanic whites."

Although his early research showed that Hispanics had a similar life expectancy to white Americans, it was soon discovered that Hispanics actually outlived them by an average of two to three years.

Hispanics also seem to survive and recover from disease more quickly than non-Hispanic whites, according to research by Dr. John Ruiz, assistant professor of psychology at the University of North Texas (UNT). "We're seeing a survival advantage across disease conditions."

Ruiz spent two years combing through fifty-eight studies of more than 4.5 million participants spanning two decades, applying complex statistical analyses, before agreeing that the Hispanic paradox really does exist. His study found an overall 17.5 percent lower risk of death for Hispanics than for other ethnic and racial groups. But it couldn't find an explanation. "I don't think there's any one factor to explain it," he says. "There are crumbs in the literature, and we're sort of piecing the crumbs together."

One of those crumbs is the "migration-selection" hypothesis: the idea that immigrants are healthier to begin with. Immigration, legal or otherwise, is a rigorous process that weeds the strong from the weak. Stamina, strength, and good health are needed to endure the ordeal.

"There are barriers to migration," Markides says. "Exams to pass. And even if they migrate illegally, there are still barriers like crossing the Rio Grande. These barriers favor healthy people."

More than one-third of the 57 million Hispanics living in the United States are immigrants. The migration selection hypothesis could explain their superior health status but doesn't explain why US-born Hispanics also outlive other groups.

Another theory that tries to explain the paradox is the "salmon-bias" hypothesis. It postulates that Hispanic immigrants return to their country of origin to die. This reverse migration would result in their exclusion from death data in the United States, making it seem as if the Hispanic population as a whole lives longer. But studies have shown that the opposite is true. Hispanic immigrants who have returned to their country of origin often come back to the United States when they fall ill so that they can be cared for by family.

Good health care certainly doesn't seem to explain why Hispanic immigrants live longer than white Americans. In Texas, the uninsured capital of the United States, more than 4.5 million people lack health insurance. Nearly two-thirds of the uninsured—more than 3 million—are Hispanic.

Lack of health insurance means a lower chance of detecting diseases like cancer, especially in the early, more treatable stages of the illness. And this is reflected in a recent study that found that Hispanics in Texas are usually diagnosed with cancer much later than white Americans. But even then, Hispanic immigrants are more likely than whites to survive cancer. It's yet another paradox.

"It's a very puzzling fact," says Dr. John S. Goodwin, a doctor at the University of Texas Medical Branch, who led the cancer study. "We found that Hispanics are less likely to get mammograms and colon cancer screening, but their survival after a cancer diagnosis is superior to non-Hispanic whites."

In 2017, a sociologist at the University of California, Irvine, called the immigrant paradox into question, particularly the idea that children raised in immigrant families have higher educational achievement compared to the children of people born in the United States. Cynthia Feliciano's research, published in the *American Sociological Review,* found that Asian immigrants to the United States were often well educated and had a higher socioeconomic status in their home countries.

"It is not just that immigrants are highly motivated and achievement-oriented because they have migrated for opportunities, but that U.S. immigrants originated from higher social class locations, providing them with a particular set of class-specific resources—a *habitus,* for example—that buttresses their children's achievement," Feliciano wrote. Those immigrant families were able to maneuver into similar social strata when they arrived in the United States.

But that's not often true for immigrants from Latin America, who have the highest rates of poverty among immigrants living in the United States. More than 30 percent of immigrants from Mexico live in poverty, compared to 14 percent of immigrants from China and 5.3 percent from the Philippines, according to data from the Center for Immigration Studies.

Most of the theories proposed to explain how immigrants living in poverty outlive American-born people, lead back to family—and, in essence, love—an idea that makes Dr. Kyriakos Markides chuckle. When asked if love is the answer to a longer life he says, "It could be. But we don't have the data to say that convincingly."

Family is a hugely important part of Hispanic culture and provides social support as well as distinct roles and duties to individuals. "The first thing you think of when you think of Hispanics is that we're a collectivistic culture," says Ruiz, the UNT professor. "The importance of family is more pronounced among Hispanics than in individualistic societies."

Ruiz points to the lower rates of infant mortality among Hispanics than non-Hispanic whites to describe how family members are actively involved in collective activities like raising children. "If you think about it, those Hispanic kids are likely to have, say, five family members who are caregivers, compared to other cultures where there's maybe only one."

Regular social interaction has been shown to keep the brain active and improve overall health. Conversely, loneliness, especially among seniors, has been linked to higher rates of depression and slower healing after surgery. "That's a pretty consistent finding in the studies," says Ruiz. "People with higher social support experience better health outcomes."

Goodwin agrees that the importance of family may lie at the heart of the Hispanic paradox and that the survival advantage might be explained by the fact that Hispanics who are sick and hospitalized are more likely to be sent home and taken care of by family, compared with other groups. "We think social support is a big factor," he says.

Hispanics don't have a monopoly on tight-knit communities. Nor are they the only immigrants to have a health status more comparable to white Americans. A "new immigrant paradox" has been observed in other immigrant populations in the United States, but it is far more apparent, and stronger, among Hispanics. This might be because they make up the largest proportion of immigrants in the United States.

About half of the foreign-born population in the United States is from Latin America. Mexican immigrants alone outnumbered all immigrants from South and East Asia in 2011, according to the Pew Research Center's Hispanic Trends Project. So even immigrants who cross the border alone are more likely to find community and cultural protection if they come from Mexico than if they come from Asia.

In Texas, Hispanics are the fastest-growing ethnic group and will outnumber the state's white population by 2020. They are expected to make up the majority of the state's population by 2042. The Census Bureau estimates that Texas is adding a quarter-million Hispanic residents a year.

Researchers have also found that immigrants in general become less healthy the longer they stay in the United States. But living in a neighborhood with a higher concentration of immigrants, even if that neighborhood is poor, provides health protection. A study by researchers at the University of Chicago in 2007 found lower rates of asthma and breathing problems among Hispanic immigrants living in communities with higher proportions of immigrants.

What a barrio may lack in wealth and safety, it may make up for in social support and love. "These are neighborhoods where you have more ethnic density," says Ruiz, referring to a higher concentration of Hispanic immigrants in one area. "Folks in these neighborhoods tend to have better health outcomes than Hispanics of the same socioeconomic status who live in less ethnically dense neighborhoods."

Love may not sound scientific—and scientists like to be taken seriously—and it's difficult to measure. But if you read between the lines of the articles published in esteemed medical journals, it's there. And it may not be as unscientific as it sounds. In the same way that poverty is proven to be bad for your health, studies have shown that loving family and social networks are good for your health.

New research could shed light on this and anything unique about the role of family in Hispanic culture. Sixteen thousand Hispanics in four cities across the United States are being interviewed in the Hispanic Community and Health Study, led by the National Institutes of Health. Importantly, the researchers will be asking questions about family structure, community involvement, and traditional Hispanic values, alongside questions about health.

Finding the key to the paradox could help us all live longer. Understanding what gives Hispanics and new immigrants a health advantage, and integrating that into health education, could benefit people of all races. But after nearly thirty years and hundreds of studies looking at the health behaviors, migration patterns, and characteristics of Hispanics, scientists still haven't solved the Hispanic paradox.

27

Has the US government banned research about gun violence?

I f you are an American man, you will probably die at least two years and two months earlier than men in other high-income countries. Men in Australia and Iceland live into their eighties. American men, on average, die at 76.

What kills them sooner? It's not heart disease or cancer. It's a combination of three things, including car crashes and drug overdoses. But the third and biggest contributor to the shortened lives of American men is guns.

Gun violence cuts more than five months off the life expectancy of American men, say researchers at the National Center for Health Statistics who compared the life expectancy of men in a dozen high-income countries.

Public health experts say that gun violence needs to be treated like a disease. If the biggest contributor to the life expectancy gap were cancer, there would be screening programs, education campaigns, and treatments developed to halt it. They worry that fear of offending Second Amendment rights advocates means gun violence is not being treated as a public health threat and that silence is killing thousands.

Some cities are starting to treat gun violence like an illness. When a Delaware city experienced a 45 percent increase in shootings in 2013, local officials called in disease detectives from the Centers for Disease Control and Prevention. Those investigators are usually tasked with studying and stopping epidemics of diseases such as meningitis and HIV or limiting the health effects of a natural disaster.

But in Wilmington, Delaware, they used the same tools they employ to curb infections to understand why gun violence was on the rise. Their work helped city officials understand who is most at risk of becoming a victim of gun violence and when to intervene to prevent shooting deaths.

Some experts say the CDC investigation of the gun violence epidemic in Delaware skirted the real issues and that federal disease detectives were fearful to study how people acquired guns and to investigate whether policies to limit access to guns would slow the epidemic.

That's because a number of murky rules have left the CDC unclear as to what it is and isn't allowed to research when it comes to guns. Some believe there's an outright ban on the agency studying gun violence. While that's not true, it often feels that way.

Understanding why requires a quick look at its history of gun research in America. From 1986 to 1996, the CDC sponsored and carried out public health research on gun violence. In 1993, it funded a study by researchers at the University of Tennessee. The researchers found that "rather than confer protection, guns kept in the home are associated with an increase in the risk of homicide by a family member or intimate acquaintance."

The National Rifle Association didn't like that. It lobbied to get rid of the CDC's Center for National Injury Prevention, and while that didn't happen, it was successful in another sense. In 1996, Congress added a few lines to the Omnibus Appropriations Bill. It said: "None of the funds made available for injury prevention and control at the Centers for Disease Control and Prevention may be used to advocate or promote gun control."

No one really knew what that meant. The addition was known as the Dickey Amendment after its author, Republican Arkansas lawmaker and lifetime NRA member Jay Dickey.

The Dickey Amendment didn't exactly ban research into gun violence, but it certainly had an impact. Just look at what happened next: Congress took the amount that the CDC had spent on researching gun violence in 1995—about $2.6 million—from the CDC's budget and said that money should be spent studying something else.

When I worked at the CDC, I asked injury prevention researchers what the Dickey Amendment meant to them. They told me they were worried about hurting their careers and losing the center money if they continued to study gun violence. They shifted their research elsewhere.

Dickey eventually changed his mind about his namesake amendment. In a *Washington Post* op-ed in 2012, he referred to himself as the "NRA's point person in Congress" and said the amendment "sent a chilling message." The op-ed was co-written by a former director of the CDC's Center for National Injury Prevention. The pair wrote: "Since the [Dickey Amendment] passed in 1996, the United States has spent about $240 million a year on traffic safety research, but there has been almost no publicly funded research on firearm injuries." That op-ed was published five months before the massacre at Sandy Hook Elementary in Connecticut, where twenty children and six adults were shot to death.

One month after the massacre, President Barack Obama issued an executive order saying that the director of the CDC "shall conduct or sponsor research into the causes of gun violence and the ways to prevent it." But the CDC is still too nervous to study gun violence. Congress didn't help: It blocked bills in 2012 and 2013 that would have provided $10 million in funding for the CDC's gun violence research, which Obama had requested.

The interjection of gun politics in health is not limited to federal agencies. Second Amendment activists in Florida supported a 2011 law that makes it illegal for Florida doctors to "ask questions concerning the ownership of a firearm" during a consultation.

The purpose of the law, they say, is to protect patient privacy. Except existing laws already protect patient privacy. What the Firearm Owners' Privacy Act does is stop doctors from asking about gun ownership and ban pediatricians from asking parents how guns are stored in the home.

A doctor charged with making sure kids are safe can lose his or her license for asking if parents own a gun safe and know how to store guns safely. Close to 1.7 million American children live in homes where guns are stored loaded or are not locked away, according to the Law Center to Prevent Gun Violence. Gun violence is the second leading cause of death of American children.

When a Florida judge issued an injunction against the Florida law in 2012, the court of appeals reversed it, saying, "The practice of good medicine does not require interrogation about irrelevant, private matters."

Guns are a relevant, public health threat, and good medicine requires honest discussions about everything from eating habits to gun ownership. By talking about deaths from driving, we've made strides in road safety through seat belts and speed limits. We could make gun ownership safer for everyone. But it's hard to treat an illness if you refuse to talk about it and the agency tasked with controlling and protecting the health of Americans is too fearful to do its job.

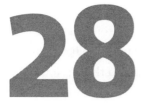

The Frackademia Scandal

Did oil and gas companies pay academics to say fracking was safe?

T imothy Considine predicted that fracking would create more than 48,000 jobs in Pennsylvania in 2009, almost 175,000 jobs in 2020, and $400 million in state and local tax revenues. Considine was professor of energy and environmental economics in the Pennsylvania State University's College of Earth and Mineral Sciences when he began his study. He co-authored it with a Penn State professor emeritus and two Penn State professors. Soon after the study began, he moved to the University of Wyoming, where he became director of its Center for Energy Economics and Public Policy.

The cover of the report and every single page thereafter bore the Penn State logo. But the report was missing one detail. Nowhere did it mention who had funded the research on fracking—that would be a consortium of gas drilling companies.

Hydraulic fracturing, better known as fracking, is the literal smashing, or fracturing, of rock, using millions of gallons of water, which is injected into the rock at high pressure along with a mixture of sand and undisclosed chemicals.

Fracking is a way of extracting oil and gas buried deep in the ground in shale rock (a type of mudstone), which wouldn't be accessible using traditional oil drilling.

Fracking is a trillion-dollar a year industry, according to the National Bureau of Economic Research. It saves Americans billions of dollars in gas prices, lowers the amount of greenhouse gas–producing coal used to make electricity, and is responsible for the generation of thousands of jobs. NO, IT DOESN'T

Just not as many jobs as Considine predicted. Considine tweaked the jobs numbers in an updated report the next year. It turned out the actual number of jobs created by the fracking industry in 2009 was fewer than his team had projected, although, in the same report, they upped the 2020 projections to nearly 212,000 new jobs.

FRACKING

The United States gets 67 percent of its natural gas and around half of its oil from fracking, according to the US Energy Information Administration. Fracking is said to have driven down the country's gas prices, made the United States less reliant on international energy sources, and on coal, which generates double the amount of carbon dioxide when used to generate electricity.

The fracking process begins with the drilling of holes hundreds or thousands of feet vertically or horizontally into the ground. Gallons of water—up to 8 million gallons and up to 40,000 gallons of chemicals—are injected into the ground at each well site. The technique was developed in the 1940s to provide access to hard to reach pockets of gas and oil, but the type of fracking performed currently, known as deep fracking, was first used in Texas in 1999.

But since its first use, there have been concerns about the impact of fracking on public health and the environment. First, there's the large amount of chemical-laced water used at each well, sometimes requiring 2,000 tanker trips to supply one site.

The amount of water used in the process is increasing. Fracking used twenty-nine times the amount of water in 2014 than in 2000, up from around 177,000 gallons per well to 5.1 million gallons, according to the US Geological Survey. As a helpful comparison, the USGS said, "an Olympic-sized swimming pool holds about 660,000 gallons."

In dry regions, this amount of water used in fracking can impact the local supply. In a 2018 study, scientists found around a third of the world's shale deposits are in arid regions and up to 40 percent of shale deposits are in places where water shortages could be worsened by fracking.

Then there are the chemicals added to the water. While they make up a very small proportion of the fluid volume—typically 0.5 to 2 percent—more than 2,000 chemicals are known to be used in what's called "frackwater," the mixture injected at high pressure into shale rock buried deep in the ground.

Chemicals are added to the water and sand mixture to decrease friction and limit corrosion. More than 600 of these additives are toxic, according to an investigation by Congress. It's hard to know which chemicals are used and where because not all states require companies to disclose which chemicals they add to their proprietary blends of frackwater. The companies say they need to keep their frackwater recipes secret from competitors.

The chemicals sometimes show up in local water supplies. In 2008, residents of Pavillion, Wyoming, complained of a foul smell to their water and a strange taste. The small town sits on the Wind River Basin, which is home to more than 180 oil and gas wells.

Residents even wondered if their strange-smelling water was to blame for some of the town's people falling sick. In 2008, they contacted the Environmental Protection Agency and in March 2009, the EPA sampled water from thirty-nine wells in the area. The next year it sampled water from forty-one locations. It found that groundwater in Pavillion was contaminated with petroleum hydrocarbons and petroleum compounds such as benzene, xylene, methylcyclohexane, naphthalene, and phenol. Benzene is a highly flammable chemical used in lighter fluid. Naphthalene is found in car exhausts and cigarette smoke.

The EPA linked the contaminants to fracking, in a 2011 report, which sparked criticism from oil and gas companies. A few years later, it transferred the investigation to state regulators, who published a series of reports that didn't reach any conclusions. Those investigations abruptly stopped.

But a former EPA scientist took the matter into his own hands. Dominic DiGiulio, at the time a scholar at Stanford School of Earth, Energy and Environmental Sciences, took publicly available data accessed through Freedom of

Information Act requests, analyzed the data and published his findings in the peer-reviewed journal *Environmental Science and Technology* in 2016.

The water in Pavillion was poisoned. The entirety of the groundwater in the area was contaminated with chemicals used in fracking, DiGiulio's study said. "We showed that groundwater contamination occurred as a result of hydraulic fracturing. It contaminated the Wind River formation," DiGiulio told reporters.

His team found that fracking waste was dumped in underground pits, which were often unlined. There was also the dumping of drilling fluids, which contained diesel and insufficient cement barriers to protect groundwater.

"It's perfectly legal to inject stimulation fluids into underground drinking water resources. This may be causing widespread impacts on drinking water resources," DiGiulio said in a Stanford University press release.

The Energy Policy Act exempts fracking from the Safe Drinking Water Act. An addition to the 2005 bill was added by then vice president Dick Cheney, a former chief executive at Halliburton. The provision prevented the EPA from investigating fracking. It was nicknamed the Halliburton loophole.

Fracking has also been found to shake the ground. Earthquakes measuring up to 4.6 M have occurred close to fracking sites in Texas, Oklahoma, Kansas, and elsewhere. It's not the fracking itself, rather an activity related to fracking that is rocking the earth. After the mixture of water, sand, and chemicals is injected into the ground, it flows back up to the surface. The wastewater has to be disposed of and one way of doing that is to inject it into underground wells. It's this activity, the injecting of wastewater into deep wells, that is causing the earthquakes.

And it's not only fracking that produces seismic shifts from wastewater disposal in subterranean wells. In fact, most of the water disposed in those underground wells comes from traditional oil drilling.

The USGS says that in Oklahoma, the state with the most induced earthquakes, "only 1-2% of the earthquakes can be linked to hydraulic fracturing operations. The remaining earthquakes are induced by wastewater disposal."

Explosions from methane leaks, worksite accidents, and air pollution with greenhouse gases are some of the side effects of fracking that oil and gas companies want to hide, activists say. The companies are using their considerable power and wealth to buy academics, so-called frackademics, who publish seemingly neutral, scientific studies that show fracking in a falsely positive light.

FRACKADEMIA

On top of the rosy picture that Timothy Considine and his fellow scientists painted of the fracking industry in their 2009 report about Pennsylvania, they issued a warning to policy makers. Burdening gas companies with a severance tax would cause fracking to decline 30 percent over two decades and would result in $880 million in lost tax revenue.

The research focused on the Marcellus Shale, which stretches throughout the northern Appalachian Basin from West Virginia through Pennsylvania to Maryland and New York. It's the largest onshore natural gas reserve in the United States, home to 262 trillion cubic feet of buried natural gas.

Considine's second report caught the eye of an advocacy organization called the Responsible Drilling Alliance, which noticed red flags in his earlier work. It wrote a letter to Penn State, which retracted Considine's original report. "We found flaws in the way the report was written and presented to the public," wrote William Easterling, dean of Penn State's College of Earth and Mineral Sciences.

Although he defended the methodology and science as "sound" and said it did "not appear to have any significant flaws," the dean chastised the scientists for featuring Penn State's logo on every page of the report, for not disclosing the study's sponsor, and for crossing the line from analysis to advocacy. "The prose in the section dealing with potential effects of a severance tax on drilling rates in Pennsylvania should be more scholarly and less advocacy minded."

Considine is one of a growing number of scientists dubbed frackademics by advocacy groups. Frackademics take money from oil and gas companies, often don't disclose their funding sources, and produce seemingly objective scientific studies that show fracking in an overwhelmingly positive light.

"When does a study on the unconventional shale gas industry become a 'shill gas study?'" wrote Steve Horn, a blogger at DeSmogBlog, which covers gas and oil companies. "The quick answer: when nearly everyone writing and peer reviewing it has close ties to the industry they're purportedly doing an 'objective' study on."

The DeSmogBlog was founded in 2006 with the aim of opposing "a well-funded and highly organized public relations campaign" that is "poisoning" the climate change debate.

Horn has meticulously covered the emergence of what he and others refer to as frackademia, uncovering the hidden connections between scientists in the academy and gas and oil companies. From questionable research by scientists at the Massachusetts Institute of Technology, the University of Texas at Austin, and the State University of New York at Buffalo, to name a few.

In May 2012, Considine was lead author of a report that said fracking was becoming safer. Published one month after the University at Buffalo opened its Shale Resources and Society Institute, critics said the report was biased and inaccurate.

Considine "and his co-authors massaged Pennsylvania Department of Environmental Protection data to support untenable claims that environmental violations by frackers are on the decline," said the Public Accountability Initiative, a nonprofit organization that investigates corporate and government corruption. It said fracking was becoming more dangerous.

The University at Buffalo was forced to issue a correction, stripping the study of its peer-reviewed designation. Then, seven months after it opened, the institute closed down. A petition signed by more than 10,000 people including faculty and students, demanded the institute be shuttered.

The university's financial disclosure policies had been "inconsistently applied," wrote university president Satish Tripathi, and this had impacted the institute's appearance of integrity and independence. There was a "cloud of uncertainty over its work." Considine's co-author Robert Watson had also worked with him on his 2009 study about fracking in Pennsylvania.

At the same time, academics at Penn State pulled out of a fracking study funded by the Marcellus Shale Coalition. Under increased scrutiny and a great deal of national press coverage, the coalition was forced to cancel its funding.

Scientists at the University of Texas at Austin, the Massachusetts Institute of Technology, and the University of Southern California are among those accused of being frackademics. A 2012 study by scientists at the University of Texas at Austin said there was no evidence of groundwater contamination from fracking. Critics said the science was deeply flawed.

There were more hidden ties. The chief scientist of that study, Charles Groat, had failed to reveal an important affiliation. He was a board member of an oil and gas company involved in fracking. "Groat earned more than double his University of Texas salary as a PXP board member in 2011—$413,900 as opposed to $173,273—and he has amassed over $1.6 million in stock during his tenure there," wrote the watchdog group, the Public Accountability Initiative.

Some universities have launched investigations into studies accused of bias and falsification. But at the University of Texas at Austin, the chair of one such investigation was himself a former board member of a multinational oil and gas company. Norman Augustine had served for nearly two decades at ConocoPhillips and Phillips Petroleum. He was also the former chair and CEO of Lockheed Martin. The university's executive vice president and provost didn't seem to mind. He said Augustine's "credentials are impeccable."

The list of frackademics might be getting longer because of funding cuts to American universities. More than $1.4 billion was cut from the State University of New York public university system between 2008 and 2011, according to SUNY officials. In 2011, lawmakers cut another $289 million from the system.

Cuts create empty spaces for the oil and gas industry to fill. "It's a growing problem across academia," said Mark Partridge, a professor of rural-urban policy at the Ohio State University. Speaking to reporters at Bloomberg, Partridge said, "Universities are so short of money, professors are under a lot of pressure to raise research funding in any manner possible."

Besides the crossing of ethical lines, the realization that scientists are human and prone to coercion and the destruction of trust in science, there are at least two more problems with the frackademia scandal.

Academic studies inform policy. The report co-authored by Considine and published under the auspices of the University at Buffalo was used as evidence to defend fracking in Pennsylvania to the House of Representatives Committee on Oversight and Government Reform. The retracted Penn State report was used to encourage policy makers not to raise taxes for gas companies.

By pushing scientists toward their agenda, gas and oil companies also push money and attention toward the questions they want answered. That means we end up with a lot of research on cheaper, quicker, more aggressive ways of getting gas out of the ground but lack sufficient research on the health and environmental impact of fracking, especially the effects on those communities who live where fracking is performed.

And it's not just frackademics who are being bought. University land is up for sale, too. In 2011, Pennsylvania governor Tom Corbett signed a bill allowing drilling for gas to take place on state university property. The previous year, the governor cut funding to the Pennsylvania State System of Higher Education by 18 percent while pocketing $1.3 million from the gas and oil industry himself, according to the National Institute on Money in State Politics, which tracks campaign finance data. The University of Texas and some universities in West Virginia lease university land to gas companies. Ohio is on track to do the same.

Frackademia can be a tricky business to investigate. It's not unusual for scientists to move back and forth between jobs in industry and jobs in academia. In fact, universities appreciate those scientists who bring real world experience to the campus. But academia is assumed to be neutral, a referee of sorts, in a playing field of uncertainty and controversy. The oil and gas industry's deep pockets and ability to buy academics and sway their research leaves the public vulnerable to misinformation and not knowing who or what to believe regarding fracking.

29

Does playing American football give players brain damage?

n June 2012, 2,138 former National Football League players filed a lawsuit against the NFL in federal court. The lawsuit was dubbed a "megalawsuit" because it consolidated eighty-one separate lawsuits from former players as well as more than 1,000 current players and their families. The megalawsuit charged that the NFL knew the long-term health risks associated with repetitive head injury and "fraudulently concealed" the impact of head trauma.

Football players, the lawsuit stated, were "at significant risk of developing long-term brain damage and cognitive decline as a result" of playing professional football. It also said the NFL's response to head trauma had been "until very recently, a concerted effort of deception and denial."

One month before the lawsuit was filed, Junior Seau, a Hall of Fame linebacker and a twenty-year veteran of the NFL, died of suicide. He was 43 years old. In his two decades playing in the NFL, Seau was never listed as having suffered a concussion. But a few years before his death he told a friend: "I've had a headache for years. I can't tell you how many concussions I had."

Family members said Seau had been depressed and irritable for months before he died. A year earlier, another NFL player, Dave Duerson, died in the same way as Seau: from a self-inflicted gunshot wound to the chest. Fifty-year-old Duerson texted his wife before he killed himself: "Please, see that my brain is given to the NFL's brain bank."

Autopsies of both men revealed brains that were scarred and riddled with abnormal bundles of protein when viewed under a microscope. A report on Seau's autopsy was released by the National Institutes of Health, the government's health research agency, which was studying the brains of professional athletes.

Two experts at the NIH verified the abnormal findings. Then they sent the brain to three independent brain experts, not disclosing who the brain belonged to. Those three experts confirmed the diagnosis: Seau had suffered from chronic traumatic encephalopathy, better known as CTE. His 43-year-old brain looked like it belonged to an elderly man suffering with Alzheimer's disease. Duerson's brain was riddled with the same pathology.

CTE is a degenerative disease of the brain that gets progressively worse. It is likely caused by repetitive brain injury such as blows to the head, although the causes of CTE are still being studied. It's a relatively new area of research that's not yet fully understood. One of the challenges of CTE is that it cannot be diagnosed in a living person. It can only be diagnosed in death when a brain autopsy is performed.

Although it might appear healthy to the naked eye, the brain of a person with CTE can sometimes look shrunken and weigh less than a healthy brain. Under the microscope is where CTE shows itself. The brain is laced with proteins called tau, specifically hyperphosphorylated tau or p-tau, which forms three kinds of protein bundles in the brain—neurofibrillary tangles, glial tangles, and neuropil threads. These protein tangles kill brain cells.

The location of those p-tau protein tangles in the brain is important because the buildup of p-tau is not unique to CTE. Patients with Alzheimer's suffer with the same p-tau tangles. But in CTE, these tangles have a particular signature. They are found in irregular clusters around small blood vessels and burrowed in the deep grooves of the brain. Repetitive trauma is thought to cause kinks in the p-tau protein, triggering it to stick to other tau proteins and form toxic clumps.

These brain changes, as well as symptoms of CTE, can occur soon after brain trauma or many years—even decades—after injury. It might even be decades before a person suffers memory loss, delusions, mood and behavior changes, suicidal ideation, and dementia.

The brain trauma believed to contribute to CTE includes everything from concussion, at the mildest end of the brain injury spectrum, to more severe brain trauma. Some brain experts are discouraging use of the term *concussion* and instead asking doctors to more precisely grade the severity of brain trauma. Brain injury can be hard to diagnose, and even trauma without immediate symptoms, such as a blackout or ringing in the ears, is thought to trigger the buildup of abnormal protein tangles in the brain.

A CTE rating scale has been developed by Dr. Ann McKee, director of the Boston University CTE Center. McKee's team divides CTE into four stages: stage 1 includes headaches and problems with concentration and attention. In stage 2, a person might suffer with depression, short-term memory loss, and anger problems. In stage 3, a person experiences cognitive impairment and problems with executive functions. Stage 4 CTE is full-blown dementia.

Looking at slices of Junior Seau's brain under the microscope, McKee said he had at least stage 2 CTE. Dave Duerson suffered stage 4 of the disease.

PUNCH DRUNK

Strange behavior in athletes whose sport exposes them to blows to the head has been recorded in the medical literature since the 1920s. In a case series of five boxers published in the October 1928 issue of the *Journal of the American Medical Association,* Dr. Harrison Martland described the men as staggering around the place acting "goofy" and "slug nutty." One man, a 38-year-old who had boxed since he was 16, suffered a left hand tremor and unsteadiness in his legs since age 23.

Martland called the boxers *punch drunk,* the term used by Americans in the 1920s to describe the "peculiar" behavior of fighters who had "taken considerable head punishment." It was the first mention of brain damage from concussions in the medical literature.

"I am of the opinion that in punch drunk there is a very definite brain injury due to single or repeated blows on the head or jaw which cause multiple concussions," wrote Martland.

Nine years later, the naval medical officer J. A. Millspaugh introduced the term *dementia pugilistica* in the *US Naval Medical Bulletin*. *Pugilistica* comes from the Latin word *pugnus*, meaning "fist" and was used perhaps as a more polite way than *punch drunk* to refer to the brain disease afflicting fighters.

The first mention of CTE appears in 1940. That's when two American psychiatrists, Dr. Karl Bowman and Dr. Abram Blau, referred to paranoia, childish behavior, aggression, poor orientation, and memory problems in boxers as CTE of pugilists. In 1949, yet another paper on strange behaviors among boxers was published, this time by British neurologist Dr. Macdonald Critchley, who also used the term *CTE* to describe the affliction.

But even Martland, back in 1928, seemed to have known he was dealing with a litigious subject of "enormous importance to the courts and to labor compensation boards." A few decades later, CTE was to become entangled with one of the biggest and wealthiest sporting institutions in the world.

It was in the 1990s that attention moved from CTE in boxers to CTE in professional football players. In October 1994, Merril Hoge, an eight-season running back with the Pittsburgh Steelers and the Chicago Bears, retired. Hoge had famously taken a knee to the head in a game, an injury that left him temporarily unable to recognize his brother or his wife. He quit football at age 29, telling journalists, "This is messing with your brain." Then he sued the Bears' doctor for not warning him about the severity of the head injuries he suffered. A jury awarded him $1.45 million.

Hoge was possibly the first NFL player to retire with a public acknowledgment that injuries to the head were his reason for quitting. But there were more to come.

As awareness grew about strange neurological symptoms in footballers, the NFL began to downplay the harms of head injuries and the possible connection between concussions and brain disease. The same year that Hoge retired, the NFL established the Mild Traumatic Brain Injury (MTBI) committee and appointed a chair who was a rheumatologist, not a neurologist. Dr. Elliot Pellman said: "Concussions are part of the profession, an occupational risk." Pellman, who himself as a team doctor let concussed players go back onto the field to play, said drug use was "a far greater problem" than concussions.

NFL commissioner Paul Tagliabue blamed journalists for the interest in head injuries among players. He said concussions were "one of these pack journalism issues . . . There is no increase in concussions, the number is relatively small . . . The problem is a journalist issue."

But evidence was growing about a possible connection between repeated head injuries and the buildup of toxic proteins in the brain. One of the first doctors to show the connection between football and the tangle of proteins jamming up the brains of pro football players thought science would help the league tackle the problem.

Bennet Omalu, a Nigerian doctor working in Pittsburgh, was squaring off against a multibillion-dollar corporation. And with inconclusive scientific evidence that football was the cause of CTE, the NFL continued to play the denial game.

In 2002, Omalu was working as a pathologist in the Allegheny County coroner's office when the body of Mike Webster arrived in his morgue. Webster was the 50-year-old Hall of Famer who had played for the Kansas City Chiefs and for fifteen seasons and 220 games with the Pittsburgh Steelers—the most in the team's history. Webster died of a heart attack in 2002 after suffering years of delusions, paranoia, depression, memory loss, and dementia.

Three years before he died, Webster filed a disability claim with the NFL Retirement Board, saying that football had caused him to suffer dementia. In October that year, the board ruled that head injuries from playing football had "totally and permanently" disabled him. Five doctors, including one working for the NFL, confirmed that Webster had suffered head injuries because of concussions.

By the time Webster arrived in Omalu's morgue, he had spent months homeless and living in a car with a broken window. After examining his heart, Omalu requested special permission to study Webster's brain. The results were stunning.

Just as Seau and Duerson's brains would show a decade later, Webster's brain was laced with tangles of toxic p-tau proteins. His was the first brain to show the microscopic changes of CTE in a football player.

Then the backlash began. After Omalu published his findings in the journal *Neurosurgery* in 2005 (science is slow), doctors from the NFL's MTBI committee (the one chaired by a rheumatologist), pushed back.

"We disagree with the assertion that Omalu et al.'s recent article actually reports a case of 'chronic traumatic encephalopathy in a National Football League (NFL) player,' " wrote Dr. Pellman and colleagues in a letter to the journal's editor. The NFL doctors said there were flaws with Omalu's findings, including the brain pathology he described, an assertion that Omalu later countered as absurd, given that he was the pathologist, not them.

The NFL doctors "urged" Omalu and his colleagues to retract their paper. Omalu refused. He went on to perform an autopsy on a second NFL player and published those findings in the same journal, with the title "Chronic Traumatic Encephalopathy in a National Football League Player: Part II."

Then he decided it would be best to continue his studies of NFL players' brains in a less public manner. "You can't go against the NFL. They will squash you," he told the PBS news show *Frontline*.

The NFL continued to refute his findings and the research of other scientists such as Dr. Ann McKee at Boston University. In 2007, when the league held its first institution-wide concussion summit, one NFL doctor told reporters: "The only scientifically valid evidence of C.E. in athletes is in boxers." Dr. Ira Casson, who was co-chair of the MTBI committee and who had called for Omalu's paper to be retracted, was referring to chronic encephalopathy.

At the same meeting, the NFL developed concussion guidelines, its first ever, according to some experts. And it launched the 88 Plan, which provided players with up to $88,000 a year for medical costs related to dementia. It was both offering support for retired players living with neurological disease and shunning any association between their illness and football.

By the time the 2012 megalawsuit was filed, the evidence linking football and CTE had piled up considerably. But there still wasn't conclusive proof that playing football causes CTE. A true link between repetitive head injuries and CTE would require a randomized controlled trial where some people suffered head injuries, some didn't, and all of the participants' brains were examined under a microscope. (They'd have to be dead for that final part.)

MONEY AND INFLUENCE:
A CONGRESSIONAL INVESTIGATION

McKee and her team were undeterred by those casting doubt on their research. But one of the main funders of McKee's research was the National Institutes of Health, and it seemed as if the NFL was trying to buy the NIH's influence.

In 2012, the NFL gave a gift of $30 million to the NIH so it could fund research into CTE. The NIH referred to it as a "no strings attached" gift. That was not entirely true.

Going through its usual processes, the NIH asked researchers to submit proposals, graded those proposals, and awarded funding to the researcher who scored highest in the merit review. That was Dr. Robert Stern, director of clinical research at Boston University's CTE Center, the one headed by Ann McKee. Since 1996, McKee and her team had established the world's largest repository of brains for studying CTE, and they were amassing evidence for the link between football and CTE.

The NFL wasn't happy with the decision. It said Stern had conflicts of interest and was biased. It wanted the scientist who had scored second best to be awarded the funds. That scientist was Dr. Richard Ellenbogen, who happened to co-chair the NFL's Head, Neck and Spine committee.

The NFL denied that it had any veto power over the NIH's decisions. But a 2016 congressional investigation titled "The National Football League's Attempt to Influence Funding Decisions at the National Institutes of Health," said otherwise.

The NFL pressured the NIH to take $16 million away from Dr. Stern and asked for it to be redirected to doctors who worked for the NFL, the congressional report said. When the NIH stated that it would not do that, the NFL responded by not funding the study, the report said, citing ESPN's reportage on the incident.

According to the report: "Despite the NFL's attempts to influence the selection of research applicants, the integrity of the peer review process was preserved and funding decisions were made solely based on the merit of the research applications." That meant taxpayers were left to pick up the bill for the study.

Among its conclusions, the report found that "the NFL did not carry out its commitment to respect the science and prioritize health and safety."

Four months after the congressional report was released, the NFL donated $100 million to support what it referred to as independent medical research in neuroscience. It said an additional $100 million had already been pledged to study CTE and other brain disorders. McKee told reporters she was skeptical about how that money would be spent. The league had funded some of her earlier work, but she told NPR, "I will be extremely surprised if any of the 100 or 200 million comes my way. The NFL directs funding only to research they approve of." She said they considered her "too damaging."

But she persisted. McKee and her team at Boston University continued to collect the brains of hundreds of former football players. In a 2017 study of 202 of these brains, McKee found 177 football players had CTE. Three of fourteen brains of those who played football only in high school had CTE. Of the fifty-three men who played college football, forty-eight had CTE. The rate was highest among NFL players: McKee found tangles of p-tau proteins and signs of CTE in the brains of 110 of the 111 men who played in the NFL.

That still wasn't sufficient to say football causes CTE. Here's why. The brains studied at McKee's CTE Center and other brain labs like it were donated by players who were worried about their mental health while they were alive. Or, they were donated by families who were concerned that a football career had harmed their loved one's brain. That can cause a sampling bias. To overcome it, scientists would have to study many more brains belonging to members of the general public who didn't play professional football.

But even without a proven causal link between football and CTE, there's evidence that the disease lives in the brain of men who play the sport professionally. Football raises the risk of suffering brain injury, which is likely to cause CTE.

The NFL publicly acknowledged a link between football and CTE in 2016, citing McKee's findings as evidence (an earlier version of McKee's 2017 brain study had shown high rates of CTE in the brains of former football players). At a meeting of the US House of Representatives' Committee on Energy and Commerce, the NFL's senior vice president for health and safety, Jeff Miller, said a link between football and CTE had been established.

But many believe the league is saying one thing and using its power and influence to quash research on brain disorders.

30

Did the US government infect people with syphilis and gonorrhea?

C hildren were infected through injections into the spine. Men were infected through sex with prostitutes who themselves had been infected with syphilis and gonorrhea by American doctors. Some men had skin scraped off their penises so that doctors could rub syphilis into the cuts. One woman, a patient in a psychiatric hospital, had pus from a gonorrhea patient injected into her eyes.

Between 1945 and 1956, 1,308 orphans, soldiers, mental health patients, prisoners, and sex workers in Guatemala were deliberately infected with syphilis and gonorrhea by American doctors. Some were given antibiotics. Many were not. At least eighty people died.

The doctors said they wanted to learn more about sexually transmitted diseases and to see if penicillin could treat syphilis. But their notes show they changed their minds about the study objectives over and over again.

The experiments were funded by the US National Institutes of Health and approved by the surgeon general. The study was never made public, but in

2005, Susan Reverby, a professor at Wellesley College, discovered documents from the study in the University of Pittsburgh library.

"I was floored," she said. Reverby was researching another set of unethical medical experiments carried out by American doctors (more on that later), when she found the papers about the Guatemala study. They were the work of the late Dr. John Cutler, a US Public Health Service doctor who led the study.

Cutler was 28 years old and a newly qualified doctor when he began his career of unethical medical experiments. In 1943, he began the two-year Terre Haute prison experiments at the Terre Haute penitentiary in Indiana. With his colleague, Dr. John F. Mahoney, Cutler deposited gonorrhea into the penises of more than 200 men incarcerated in the Indiana prison. Both men were working on behalf of the US military, which wanted to test treatments that might prevent and treat gonorrhea in soldiers returning from combat.

The prisoners in Indiana were made aware of the experiments before they were infected. Prisoners in Guatemala were not. Academic institutions and government agencies in the United States knew about the Guatemala study—it was funded by the National Institutes of Health after all—and knew that study participants did not give their consent. Some of the men were treated with antibiotics, some were left to let the disease run its course. According to surviving records, at least one person died from the infection.

Cutler relocated his experiments from the Indiana prison to Guatemala, where prostitution was legal, and he favored testing gonorrhea prophylactics on people who had been infected through sex, instead of infected by scientists. In his notes, Cutler and his colleagues wrote of the prostitutes they paid to have sex with men in Guatemala City's Central Penitentiary. Reverby, who discovered Cutler's notes in the library at the University of Pittsburgh wrote that "the researchers actually timed how long they spent with the prostitutes and thought they acted 'like rabbits.'"

In 2016, a judge dismissed a lawsuit filed by 842 victims of the Guatemala studies and their family members. The $1 billion lawsuit alleged that Johns Hopkins University and another US institution, the Rockefeller Foundation, helped "design, support, encourage and finance" the study. Both institutions deny involvement with the experiments.

In 2010, President Barack Obama called Guatemala's president Alvaro Colom to apologize. An official statement was released by Secretary of State Hillary Clinton and Health and Human Services Secretary Kathleen Sebelius.

The Guatemala study wasn't the only set of experiments the US government had to apologize for, nor was it Cutler's last foray into abusing poor people of color. In 1997, President Bill Clinton said sorry to American survivors of unethical medical research funded and carried out by doctors working for the government, including Cutler.

From 1932 to 1972, 399 African American men, mostly sharecroppers from Macon County, Alabama, were deliberately left untreated with syphilis. Even when penicillin became the standard treatment for syphilis in 1947, the men were not told they had the infection. Instead, they were told they had "bad blood" and that they were being offered the best possible care. In reality, US Public Health Service doctors experimented on the men as they grew sicker. By the end of the study, 128 men had died from syphilis and its complications. At least forty of their wives were infected and nineteen of their children were born with syphilis.

It wasn't just inhumane, it was hypocritical. While the government was conducting unethical research on its own citizens, it was prosecuting Nazi doctors in the Nuremberg trials. Those military tribunals took place in the 1940s in Germany. The Allied Forces, including the United States and the United Kingdom, prosecuted sixteen doctors for experimenting on prisoners in concentration camps. Seven of the doctors were executed for crimes against humanity.

From this horror came the Nuremberg Code and the Helsinki Declaration, written to protect those who participate in medical studies. The Tuskegee scandal also spurred lawmakers to pass legislation protecting the rights of research participants and to ensure that similar atrocities could never occur again.

Cutler defended his experiments until his death in 2003. "The Tuskegee study has been grossly misunderstood and misrepresented this way," he said to reporters in 1993. Cutler argued that the experiments "were actually to improve the quality of care for the black community . . . And of course I was bitterly opposed to killing off the study for obvious reasons."

The Tuskegee and Guatemala studies are just two examples from a long list of unethical medical studies. There are the elderly patients at the Brooklyn

Jewish Chronic Disease Hospital, who were injected with cancer cells in the 1960s so that researchers could learn about the development of tumors. There are the children at the Willowbrook State School for Children with Mental Retardation in New York City, who were infected with hepatitis from 1956 to 1971 so that experimental treatments could be tested.

Some doctors refer to these decades as "medicine's dark chapter." But it's a chapter that should not be buried in history books. In fact, the history of medicine, going much further back than the twentieth century, is filled with nonconsensual experimentation on vulnerable people.

The effects of these unethical experiments are felt to this day. Public health experts blame a 2014 outbreak of tuberculosis in Marion, Alabama, on the government's history of unethical medical research. (In February 2015, the rate of tuberculosis in Marion was higher than the rates in India, Haiti, and Kenya.)

Marion is a two-hour drive from Tuskegee. A deep distrust of doctors and the medical establishment means some people sick with tuberculosis in Marion have been reluctant to seek help, which is one reason the outbreak spread for years. Even people who weren't alive when the Tuskegee study was stopped in 1973 have heard stories of the trial and remember being warned not to trust doctors.

The lawsuit filed by survivors of the Guatemala studies is a reminder that unethical medical experiments have occurred in recent history and that the consequences are still felt by many across the world.

31

Does talcum powder cause ovarian cancer?

Wholesome, pure, the smell of newborns. Baby powder has gone from innocent beauty product to suspect carcinogen and become the fodder of late-night legal infomercials and million-dollar lawsuits.

Talc has been used as a hygiene and cosmetic product for millennia, with evidence of its popularity among ancient Egyptians. It's a naturally occurring mineral—the softest mineral on the planet—and is mined from the earth in more than forty countries. It's used in the production of ceramics, paper, as a coating on candies to stop them from sticking to one another, and of course in baby powder.

Talc is made of oxygen, silicon, water, and magnesium but can contain trace amounts of titanium and even asbestos, a known carcinogen. Asbestos and talc are often mined near each other, which is why one can contaminate the other. Like talc, asbestos is a naturally occurring mineral containing silicon.

Johnson & Johnson began selling talc in 1894 as a way to soothe the irritation caused by their bandages. Customers loved the product and started using it to treat diaper rash, leading to the launch of Johnson's Toilet & Baby Powder.

Nowadays, Johnson & Johnson makes more money off its medicines, but its brand is almost synonymous with Johnson's Baby Powder, used by people of all ages to keep skin dry, prevent chafing, and absorb odors.

In July 2018, the company was ordered to pay close to $4.7 billion in damages to twenty-two women by a jury in Missouri. The jurors ruled in favor of the women, who said Johnson's Baby Powder caused them to develop ovarian cancer. Six of the women had died from the cancer.

The women claimed the baby powder contained asbestos and that the company concealed evidence of the asbestos for decades. In one of the earliest lawsuits against the company, a 52-year-old Texas woman, Darlene Coker, accused the company's "poison talc" for causing her mesothelioma, a cancer of the membranes that cover the abdomen and chest. She said the talc was contaminated with asbestos. But Johnson & Johnson denied that claim. Coker dropped the lawsuit. She died in 2009 after a twelve-year battle with cancer.

A Reuters investigation in December 2018 declared, "Johnson and Johnson knew for decades that asbestos lurked in its Baby Powder." Internal company memos were revealed after Coker's death, as thousands more women began suing Johnson & Johnson, claiming the talcum powder itself, not contamination with asbestos, is responsible for their cancers. Other companies that sell talcum powder, such as Gold Bond, are facing similar lawsuits. The Reuters investigation said Johnson & Johnson told the Food and Drug Administration that asbestos had not been detected in its talc.

The company lied. It didn't tell the agency that at least three tests by three different labs from 1972 to 1975 had found asbestos in its talc—in one case at levels reported as "rather high," wrote Reuters journalist Lisa Girion. There was also the omission of a 1972 lab note written by a University of Minnesota professor who tested Johnson & Johnson's Shower to Shower product. "Incontrovertible asbestos," wrote the professor.

The women who testified in the Missouri court case described the many ways they used talcum powder. Some said they sprinkled it inside their underwear, directly on their genital area, and even on sanitary towels and tampons.

That's a major concern if talc-based products contain asbestos, since asbestos causes mesothelioma and cancers of the lungs, ovaries, and larynx, according to the International Agency for Research on Cancer.

But asbestos isn't always naturally present in talc, and since 1973, when the FDA introduced a new standard, talc products have to be tested and declared asbestos-free.

In 1976, three years after the new FDA standard, ten out of nineteen talcum powders tested by researchers at Mount Sinai Hospital were found to contain asbestos fibers. Johnson & Johnson's Baby Powder was not one of them. The product that contained the highest concentration of asbestos was ZBT Baby Powder with Baby Oil. Coty, Yardley, and Faberge powders tested positive.

The news damaged the wholesome image of baby powders and cosmetics. Until Mount Sinai was forced to retract some of its findings when other labs could not confirm the results. They said the tests for asbestos were not reliable and sometimes produced false positives—and false negatives.

Since then, some lawyers have argued that asbestos was found in a Vermont talc mine used by Johnson & Johnson. In the Missouri court case, the plaintiffs' lawyer, Mark Lanier, told the court that the pharmaceutical company concealed evidence of asbestos in its talc products. He said Johnson & Johnson rigged laboratory tests to show its products were asbestos-free when they were not.

Internal Johnson & Johnson memos unsealed in lawsuits include a handwritten note from a Johnson & Johnson executive dated 1973. In the memo, the executive asks the question: if Johnson & Johnson Baby Powder contained 1 percent asbestos, how much would a baby inhale when being dusted with the powder? Calculations scribbled on the memo show the amount would be less than the legal limit at the time.

A memo dated two months later says, "Occasionally, sub-trace quantities of tremolite or actinolite are identifiable (optical Microscope) and these might be classified as asbestos fiber." Indeed, tremolite and actinolite are types of asbestos.

But lawyers for women suing the company argue that these memos demonstrate that Johnson & Johnson had some idea that their Baby Powder contained a known carcinogen. Johnson & Johnson maintains that its Baby Powder does not contain asbestos, and some juries agree. In 2017, a woman in California who claimed she developed mesothelioma because she had used Johnson's Baby Powder, lost her case.

Another group of women suing Johnson & Johnson say the talc itself, not contamination with asbestos, caused their cancers. There are three reasons the link between talc and ovarian cancers was first proposed. First, talc is chemically similar to asbestos. Second, there are similarities between ovarian cancers and mesotheliomas, the kind of cancer caused by asbestos. And third, scientists looking at cancers under a microscope have found talc particles inside ovarian tumors.

One of the first studies looking at the possible connection between talc and cancers of the human female reproductive tract was published in 1971 by a group of Welsh cancer scientists in the *Journal of Obstetrics and Gynaecology*. They looked at tumors of the ovaries and cervix and found that "in both conditions talc particles were found deeply embedded within the tumour tissue."

Talc particles likely migrated up the female genital tract, a hypothesis backed up by studies that show particles the size of talc can move from the vagina, up through the uterus, along the fallopian tubes, and to the ovaries.

But the presence of talc in the tumors wasn't proof that talc caused the tumors, the Welsh scientists cautioned. They concluded that it wasn't possible to "incriminate talc as a primary cause" of cancer based on their findings alone.

Their research began a series of studies looking for a link between talc and genital cancers. In 1982, a doctor at Harvard published a study in the journal of the American Cancer Society. Dr. Daniel Cramer looked at the medical records of 215 women in Boston who were diagnosed with ovarian cancer between 1978 and 1981 and compared them with 215 women who were similar to them in age, race, and location but who didn't have ovarian cancer.

This type of observational study is called a case control study, and it can be used to look at the relationship between a risk factor—in this case, talc—and a disease—in this case, ovarian cancer. A case control study cannot say that a risk factor causes a disease. But by comparing the talc use of women who have the disease with women who don't, scientists can determine if women exposed to talc have higher or lower odds of developing cancer.

Cramer's study found ninety-two women with ovarian cancer regularly used talcum powder, either sprinkling it on their sanitary towels, or directly onto their genital area, compared with sixty-one of the controls—the women who didn't have cancer. Cramer took into account other factors that influence the likelihood of a woman developing ovarian cancer, such as menopause, and how many times a woman has been pregnant. Adjusting for those factors, he found women who used talcum powder had a higher risk of developing ovarian cancer.

Cramer doubled the size of his study in 1999, when he looked at 563 women with ovarian cancer and 523 women who did not have cancer. Comparing their talcum powder use, Cramer found women with ovarian cancer were more likely to have used talcum powder, compared to those women who were cancer-free. Forty-five percent of women with cancer used talc, compared to 36 percent of controls.

"We conclude that there is a significant association between the use of talc in genital hygiene and risk of epithelial ovarian cancer," he wrote. Adding: "When viewed in perspective of published data on this association, warrants more formal public health warnings."

Since then, some companies have added warnings on their labels. "Frequent application of talcum powder in the female genital area may increase the risk of ovarian cancer," says the label on Assured's Shower & Bath Absorbent Body Powder. "Intended for external use only."

Does this mean the company agrees that talcum powder can cause ovarian cancer? If only the science was so clear cut. Hundreds of studies on talc and cancer have produced a mixed bag of results. Some scientists, like Cramer, found higher odds of talc use among women with cancer, while others found there was no difference. Those that show a link postulate that talc particles could cause irritation and inflammation, precursors to tumor development. Hormones such as estrogen may have a part to play in any potential connection. Talc is considered inert, meaning it's not an irritant, but studies in mice showed that pregnant mice, with higher levels of estrogen, were more likely to have an inflammatory response to usually inert materials.

A 2014 study by researchers working on the Women's Health Initiative Observational Study looked at more than 61,000 women over a period of twelve years. Unlike a case control study, which looks back at people's exposure to a risk factor, this study was a prospective one, meaning the researchers selected a group of women and followed them over time, watching to see who got sick and trying to understand why. The study found using talcum powder on the genitals was not associated with a higher risk of developing ovarian cancer.

Researchers have also looked at condoms, diaphragms, and surgical gloves, which used to be routinely dusted with talc, and found no link between a person's exposure to these items and cancer risk. In fact, a medical procedure to stop the collection of fluid in the lung cavity uses talc to stick the lining of the lung to the lining of the inner chest wall to close the space where liquid could pool. The procedure, known as pleurodesis, has been found not to increase the risk of cancer.

But it seems for every study showing talcum powder use is not associated with a risk of cancer, there's a study that says it is. There are a number of weaknesses to most of the studies, including their reliance on a woman's memory and ability to remember when, how, and for how long she used baby powder. Which might be why the dozens of lawsuits brought against talcum powder manufacturers have gone both ways, ruling in favor of companies like Johnson & Johnson some of the time, and ruling in favor of the women who say baby powder caused their cancer at other times. In 2018, two Canadian government agencies, including Canada's premier public health agency, said talcum powder should be kept away from children's faces to avoid them inhaling the dust, and women should avoid using it on their genitals because "they may cause cancer."

Cancer causes are notoriously hard to investigate and prove. While courtroom juries have issued verdicts in the dozens, the scientific jury is still out.

32

Does infection with Ebola cause lifelong symptoms?

Josephine Karwah stepped out of the Ebola treatment unit and cradled her pregnant belly. She had hobbled into the white tent two weeks earlier, during August of 2014, her knees burning with pain and threatening to buckle every fourth step.

Josephine's mother had died in the Ebola treatment unit. Her body had been carried away in a white body bag that nurses had prepared with her name written neatly on the side. Her father, too, had died from Ebola, as did her aunt and uncle. But Josephine and her unborn child were survivors. She decided she would name the baby Miracle.

Then the nightmares began. Back at home in her village, Smell No Taste, an hour's drive east of the Liberian capital, Josephine dreamt of the family members she had lost to Ebola and the horrors of the treatment unit.

Throbbing headaches interrupted her dreams, and her hips and knees ached as she tried to fall back to sleep. During the day she helped her older sister make soap to sell at the market. But her right eye burned, and her left eye made the world appear cloudy, as if drops of dew had settled on a camera lens. At the money changer's booth, she walked away with the wrong change, unable to recall how many Liberian dollars were in her purse when she left the house.

Josephine is one of Liberia's 1,500 Ebola survivors. Like Josephine, many today suffer memory loss, joint pains, muscle aches, and eye problems. These are not isolated anecdotes and vague reports. In February 2016, reporting the first findings from the largest-ever study of Ebola survivors at a conference in Boston, Mosoka Fallah, an epidemiologist from Liberia, said more than half of the patients who lived through an acute attack later reported muscle and joint problems. Approximately one year after Ebola infection, two-thirds had neurological difficulties and 60 percent reported eye problems.

Doctors began referring to this constellation of symptoms as post-Ebola syndrome as early as fall 2014, when the World Health Organization sent a team of researchers to Sierra Leone. Half of the Ebola survivors they met reported eye problems, including blindness. And this has happened before. Following small Ebola outbreaks in east and central Africa in the last twenty years, survivors suffered joint pains, muscle aches, and eye problems serious enough to prevent many from working.

But these were limited episodes of the disease and small groups of survivors. The 2014–16 west African Ebola epidemic has left 17,000 survivors at risk of post-Ebola syndrome. Like Josephine, they stepped out of treatment units and stepped into an uncertain future. There is one thing that experts and patients do know: Ebola is not over.

Fallah's office sits at one end of a long corridor in the John F. Kennedy Medical Center in Monrovia. A Harvard-trained epidemiologist, he grew up in one of Liberia's largest slums and was deep in the trenches as part of the Ebola response. Now he is at the helm of the largest-ever study of Ebola survivors. When Fallah talks about Ebola he often refers to the epidemic as a pitched battle and then quickly returns to more medical language. "At the height of the war, er, outbreak," he says, researchers set in motion a project that led to his survivor research.

To test experimental vaccines and other treatments, a coalition was formed between the National Institutes of Health in the United States and the Liberian Ministry of Health and Social Welfare called the Partnership for Research on Ebola Vaccines in Liberia (PREVAIL).

By the time the initial vaccine safety tests were completed, however, Liberia's epidemic was slowing down. The number of people becoming infected with Ebola was far fewer than expected, so the first study, PREVAIL I, was scaled back to test only for vaccine safety and immune response and not the vaccine's ability to prevent Ebola. Instead, PREVAIL scientists shifted resources to Ebola's aftereffects. Reports were coming in from across west Africa of patients who survived the disease but suffered physical and psychological problems. That is when Fallah got involved. He was appointed principal investigator for the study in Liberia and switched his focus from the Ebola response to Ebola survivors.

On a Wednesday afternoon, two days before Christmas, Fallah flicked through a patient file at the Kennedy Medical Center. He had overseen the refurbishment of the building's second floor, which was now entirely dedicated to the Ebola survivor study. Outside his office and stretching up the corridor, men and women sat in chairs that lined the walls waiting to be seen by medical staff.

Since the Ebola survivor study was launched in Liberia in 2015, more than 1,000 of the country's 1,500 Ebola survivors have agreed to take part. Their health will be monitored at semiannual checkups for five years. Each survivor is asked to bring four friends or relatives to one of the study's three sites. These are people with whom the patients have close contact but who were not infected with Ebola. Fallah says he hopes to enroll 6,000 close contacts who will serve as controls, helping researchers separate the health problems that are part of post-Ebola syndrome from those experienced by the general population in Liberia.

When Fallah presented the first findings from the study in 2016, he had grim numbers: 60 percent of the approximately 1,000 virus survivors in the study reported eye problems, 53 percent said they suffered muscle aches and joint pain, and 68 percent reported neurological problems. When Fallah's team looked more closely at those who said they had eye problems, they found 10 percent had uveitis, a swelling of the middle layer of tissue in the eye wall. The eye problems drew his attention early in the research. "We saw as the war went on—I mean, the epidemic went on—that there were different manifestations among survivors and that would drive us to do more in-depth sub-studies," he says. Those secondary investigations are part of PREVAIL III. "It was clear the first PREVAIL III sub-study had to focus on the eye."

Fallah looked to previous studies of Ebola survivors dating back to the 1990s and found that many people described eye problems in the convalescent phase. Following an outbreak in the Democratic Republic of the Congo in 1995, twenty survivors were examined over three months. Four were found to have eye pain, sensitivity to light, loss of visual acuity, and uveitis up to ten weeks after infection. After an outbreak in Uganda in 2007, forty-nine survivors were followed for more than two years. As well as memory loss, joint pain, sleep disorders, and hearing loss, survivors reported blurred vision and pain behind the eyes. More recently a study of eight patients who were treated for Ebola in US hospitals found that all suffered various symptoms of post-Ebola syndrome up to four months after leaving the hospital. Six had psychological problems including depression, anxiety, and memory loss, and five suffered eye problems including blurred vision and eye pain. There was no doubt the syndrome was real. But the existing data offered little explanation for how the virus can cause these problems.

This kind of confusion has happened before, with another virus: HIV. Back in the 1980s when researchers were presented with this new health threat, they tried to understand this novel retrovirus by applying what they knew about other diseases. The same process is happening with Ebola, says Avindra Nath, a neurologist and scientist at the NIH who works closely with Fallah.

Nath has spent the better part of three decades studying infections of the brain. Although Ebola is not a retrovirus like HIV, Nath believes that years of research invested in studying HIV and the body's response to the infection have jump-started our understanding of how Ebola affects the nervous system. "Ebola has benefited from HIV research. A lot of us involved with Ebola made our careers with HIV so we are quickly adapting our knowledge and techniques to studying these patients," he says.

Nath wonders if the neurologic symptoms in Ebola survivors are a direct result of the virus or, instead, triggered by the immune system's response to the infection. HIV, for instance, infects immune cells called macrophages in the brain, prompting the release of cytokines, small proteins that are toxic to nerve cells. Studies in monkeys have shown that Ebola also infects macrophages. Ebola also can trigger a massive "cytokine storm"—cytokines are chemical messengers between cells, highly active during an immune attack—

causing veins to leak and burst. That can cause hemorrhaging throughout the body, including the brain, which could explain the memory problems, headaches, and movement disorders Nath has seen in Ebola survivors during his visits to Liberia.

As the neurologist looks to HIV for clues to how Ebola affects the brain, others turn to different viruses to understand another symptom: the extreme fatigue in Ebola survivors. Studies have shown that up to a quarter of patients with the dengue fever virus and close to 40 percent of Epstein-Barr virus patients suffer fatigue after the acute illness. Inflammatory cytokines may be to blame. They can act on receptors in the brain causing postinfection fatigue and loss of appetite.

Painful joints seem to be one of the more common symptoms of post-Ebola syndrome. In a study of survivors of the 1995 Congo outbreak, almost two-thirds experienced joint pain two years after infection, and one-third of a Ugandan outbreak's survivors suffered from joint pain two years later.

Lumps of immune system proteins that sit inside a joint like the hip or shoulder could cause irritation and swelling. Other components of the immune system, including antibodies, could explain or even act as a surrogate marker for joint pain. After the 1995 Congo outbreak, survivors who complained of painful joints were found to have higher antibody levels, compared with survivors who did not report joint pain. Another protein might be at work in pain, too. D-dimers, small chunks of protein that break off from blood clots, have been linked to joint pain in people recovering from other infections. Patients suffering joint pain after infection with the bacteria *Neisseria meningitidis* had high levels of D-dimers in their blood. Studies looking for D-dimer–level changes have not been done on Ebola survivors.

As for the eye disease seen in many Ebola survivors, experts say it too could be a result of the immune response to Ebola. Or, more ominously, the virus could be replicating in the eye long after it has been cleared from the blood. The eyeball offers a safe place for the virus to hide out, away from detection and interference by the immune system. In one survivor the eyeball was found teeming with Ebola. In October 2014 an American physician, Ian Crozier, fell sick with Ebola while working in Sierra Leone. Less than two months after he was discharged from a US hospital, he felt pain in his left eye and noticed that its color had changed from blue to green. When doctors inserted a needle into Crozier's eye, they found more copies of the virus than had been in his blood when he was close to death weeks earlier.

The eyeball is not the only hiding place for Ebola. The testes, central nervous system, and joint cartilage can act as sanctuary sites for a number of pathogens, including HIV. These vital structures are at risk of collateral damage when the immune system wages war on foreign invaders. So to protect themselves from the inflammatory response, they have adapted clever mechanisms, including immune-suppressing molecules and physical barriers. These protective measures make them great hiding spots for viruses. Hidden reservoirs could explain how Pauline Cafferkey, a Scottish nurse who recovered from Ebola, fell sick nine months after her blood tested negative for the virus and again a year after she was first infected.

The testes could also account for why Ebola persists in the semen of some survivors months after they are free of symptoms. At the beginning of the west African outbreak, the WHO cautioned people to practice safe sex for at least three months after their blood tested negative for Ebola. That advice was based on the 1995 Congo episode, where the virus was found in the semen of survivors eighty-two days after symptom onset.

But during the west African epidemic, Ebola virus lived in the semen of some survivors for a much longer time, more than a year after acute infection. At the conference in Boston, Fallah reinforced these findings, saying the virus was found in the semen of Liberian Ebola survivors eighteen months after infection. In some men the virus disappeared from the semen and then reappeared over the course of the year. (The WHO now advises male Ebola patients to practice safe sex for a year and get their semen tested repeatedly.)

In his Monrovia office, Fallah has a patient file that belongs to a woman whose son died of Ebola in November 2015. The family reported no contact with anyone sick with Ebola or any survivors, but Fallah believes otherwise. He thinks the mother may have had sex with a survivor, not realized that she was sick with Ebola, and passed the infection to her son.

It would not be the first time Fallah had investigated a case of Ebola that was likely transmitted via sex. In March 2015 a woman who died from Ebola was found to have had sex with a man who had been discharged from an Ebola treatment unit six months earlier. Blood samples from the man tested negative for Ebola, but a semen sample tested positive.

Fallah furrows his brow when talking about the woman who contracted Ebola from a survivor. That the virus can persist after many symptoms stop—even after a patient's blood appears clear—makes him anxious for two reasons: If Ebola hides out in people who seem healthy, only to reappear from compartments deep within the body to make them sick and potentially contagious, it could spark more outbreaks.

But finding the viral genome or bits of viral RNA in the bodily fluids of survivors does not prove they are contagious, he adds. What really worries Fallah is the stigma these new findings place on survivors. "It's bad enough with post-Ebola syndrome that they have these symptoms we can't explain—and for who knows how long," he says. "Survivors are going through enough. Now imagine people are scared of them for fear of catching the virus."

A few days after Josephine left the Ebola treatment unit in Monrovia, while she was sleeping in her bed in Smell No Taste, she woke just after midnight. This time it was not nightmares or headaches, it was cramping in her abdomen. She rose to use the bathroom, and when she wiped herself she saw blood on the tissue. Then her water broke. She called for her older sister. "Ophelia!" They phoned for an ambulance but were told none were available. So they called a radio station in Monrovia for help. No one came.

Josephine paced up and down her bedroom, stopping to press her palms against the wall when it felt like her stomach was tearing. At 5 a.m., she wrapped herself in a maroon lapa, a traditional Liberian saronglike fabric, and staggered out of the house. If help would not come to her, she would find help on the streets. The village was asleep, sunrise still an hour away. Josephine walked alongside her house, clutching the walls to steady herself. As she screamed, women came out of their houses. "Help me, please help me," she cried.

But no one would come near her, fearful of touching the woman who had left the Ebola treatment unit only a few days before. When she reached the light green house at the corner of the dirt road, Josephine could no longer walk. She fell to the ground, her back against the wall, and felt the baby between her legs.

Five women approached, unwrapping their lapas as they walked. They formed a semicircle around her so the male onlookers could not watch her give birth. Josephine pushed and screamed, and Miracle was born. What a chubby boy, she thought, lifting the silent child to her chest. But Miracle was not breathing.

No one would touch Josephine. The women stared as she rocked her baby and sobbed into her chest. Only her brother came close to her. He took Miracle from her arms and wrapped the baby and placenta in a yellow towel, ready for burial.

Josephine's mother had been a midwife before she died of Ebola. "Why isn't she here to help me now?" Josephine wondered. In the weeks that followed, there were more questions: Did Ebola kill Miracle or was it because nobody would help? Would the baby have lived if an ambulance had come? Was the virus still lurking in her body, and would it harm any future pregnancies?

On visits to the Kennedy Medical Center for her survivor study appointments, Josephine asks Fallah these same questions. One afternoon she sits in Fallah's office wearing an off-the-shoulder leopard print shirt and a matching head wrap waiting for his response.

Fallah worries the uterus may be another sanctuary site for Ebola, offering the virus a safe place to hide. Then he wonders if the stress of being an Ebola survivor can cause a woman to give birth to a stillborn baby in the street with people watching but no one helping. He thinks, "When you can no longer sell soap in the market, when you have to wrap your money in tissue to buy vegetables, when your boyfriend stops loving you because you are an Ebola survivor—What impact does that have on a person's body? What could that do to their unborn child?"

This is what goes through his mind, but when Josephine asks, he says: "I don't know, Josephine. We are trying to find out."

33

Are older adults at higher risk of contracting sexually transmitted infections?

A s soon as she wakes up, Helen Goldenberg lines up her pills: twenty-three of them that she takes in four bouts over the course of the day. First, she takes her acid reflux pill, then the pills that control her blood pressure. After breakfast, she takes her HIV pill: a big blue tablet to keep the virus in check. Goldenberg is in her seventies and has lived with HIV for over thirty years.

Sexually transmitted infections, including HIV, are often conflated with youth. But more people, like Goldenberg, are living with HIV into their sixties and seventies thanks to a cocktail of medications that have drastically improved survival. One in four people living with the virus in the United States is older than 55. Not only are people living longer with HIV, they're becoming infected later in life. Nearly half of all Americans diagnosed with HIV in 2015 were aged 50 and over.

While navigating the screen on her iPhone, Goldenberg lists three close friends in Dallas who are in their fifties and sixties and who were recently diagnosed with HIV. One of them tested positive at the age of 69.

Rates of sexually transmitted infections, including HIV, have increased in the over-65 age group in recent years. Chlamydia rates nearly doubled among Americans ages 55 to 64 between 2012 and 2016, and gonorrhea cases rose 164 percent in the over-55 age group between 2014 and 2018, according to the Centers for Disease Control and Prevention.

Older people are having sex. Lots of sex. And some of it is the unprotected kind that puts them at risk for sexually transmitted infections, including HIV, syphilis, gonorrhea, and others.

But it seems that we're uncomfortable talking about the sex lives of older adults. Even the World Health Organization in a recent report confessed to collecting sexual health data only for people up to the age of 49. The false assumption that physical intimacy declines at age 50 isn't limited to the medical establishment—it's common throughout society.

In reality, more than half of people over the age of 65 are having sex, according to a study by the University of Chicago Pritzker School of Medicine. About one in four of those over the age of 75 are sexually active.

Assumptions are dangerous, and denial can fuel epidemics. A society ambivalent to the sexual health needs of older people is far removed from reality. Doctors who assume that their older patients are not sexually active are denying them the sexual health information that could save their lives.

Dr. Louis Sloan isn't so bashful. At his clinics in downtown Dallas, the infectious diseases specialist makes sure that sexual health information is available for the entire spectrum of his patient population.

Sloan is especially concerned about the number of older patients who are presenting with primary syphilis, a bacterial infection that is often asymptomatic. Diseases that don't cause symptoms can go undiagnosed for a long time if a person isn't having regular sexual health checkups.

Gonorrhea infections increased more than 90 percent, syphilis cases rose more than 60 percent, and chlamydia by more than 50 percent among those over the age of 65 during 2010–2014.

That's a problem because having one sexually transmitted infection puts you at risk of getting another one—especially HIV. Lesions, like the ones caused by syphilis and herpes, are easy entry points for the virus, and inflammation caused by other sexually transmitted infections also facilitates transmission of HIV.

People already living with HIV are five times as likely to transmit the virus when they're infected with another sexually transmitted infection. Syphilis isn't the only sexually transmitted infection that's going undiagnosed for long periods of time—it's estimated that one in five Americans with HIV aren't aware of their status.

That number could be even higher for older adults. While older adults are less likely to have multiple sexual partners than young people, the majority are sexually active. Sloan says high divorce rates and the increasing number of people living longer with HIV are contributing to the rising rates of infection.

But only 22 percent of women and 38 percent of men over the age of 50 said they had discussed sex with their doctor, according to the government's National Social Life, Health, and Aging Project. If doctors aren't considering that their older patients are having sex, they're less likely to test them for sexually transmitted infections or refer them to specialists like Sloan.

"That dialogue needs to take place," said Dr. Clinton Haley, an infectious disease doctor at Baylor University Medical Center in Dallas. "What I'm seeing is older people referred to me with subtle symptoms. They'll say, 'Oh, I'm suddenly having lots of yeast infections and I never used to get yeast infections.' And the first thing I do is test for HIV, and it comes back positive, and HIV didn't even cross their minds once."

This phenomenon explains why older adults with HIV are more likely to be diagnosed with late-stage disease, compared to younger adults. That can make it harder to treat the virus and leaves them open to passing on the virus unknowingly.

Older adults face a higher risk of heart disease, and HIV increases that risk.

"HIV causes chronic inflammation that puts you at an increased risk of getting heart disease," said Haley. "HIV as well as the meds for HIV can also cause bone density loss."

Diseases such as rectal cancers and lymphomas are more likely to occur in people with HIV. That means doctors need to screen older adults with HIV for these diseases. They also need to keep an eye on the sometimes overwhelming number of pills that older people take.

Some senior centers are struggling with the idea that their clients are having sex. Ann Wilder, a social worker at the University of North Texas who specializes in the well-being of older adults, approached a string of well-known senior centers and asked if she could discuss the issues of sexual health, sexuality, and dating in older adults. Her request was met with a resolute "no." One director eventually agreed to talk to her, but only if she could remain anonymous.

Their reticence to discuss the issue halted Wilder's graduate research on the sexual health of older adults. But her colleague, Dr. Iftekhar Amin, had another idea. He accessed government data from a nationwide survey on societal change and used that to study the sex lives of older adults.

He found that nearly three-quarters of sexually active people over the age of 55 were engaging in sexually risky behavior, like not using condoms during sex. Older women, in particular, were less empowered to negotiate safer sex in their relationships. Amin found that many stopped using condoms after menopause, indicating that birth control, rather than infectious diseases, had been their priority.

Vulnerability to sexually transmitted infections increases as we age. For women, the lining of the vagina thins and offers less protection against viruses and bacteria. In both sexes, the immune system slows so that the body is less resilient in its fight against microbes.

In addition to biology, Amin says society's archaic perception of older adults and sexuality is to blame for the rising rates of sexually transmitted infections in the over-55 age group. "We have all of these statistics out there, but no one's really talking about the issue," he says. "It's as if people just don't want to consider that their grandparents are having sex."

But today's grandparents are children of the sexual revolution—a revolution that's often credited with the advent of the contraceptive pill. The sexual education they received as young people in the 1960s and 1970s was focused more on birth control and biology and less on infectious diseases.

The next wave of sexual health education came in the 1980s, with the devastation of the AIDS epidemic. Those early AIDS campaigns were mainly targeted at young gay men; many people, now in their sixties or older, felt that AIDS education was not meant for them, especially women. That was the case with Goldenberg. "Me and my girlfriends didn't think AIDS was something that could happen to us. I was living in San Francisco back then, but AIDS was something that happened to other people, not us women."

In 1984, Goldenberg was living in San Francisco and working her way up the corporate ladder. A hard-working vice president at Bank of America, she went to the doctor's office because of a scalding cup of coffee. She thought the coffee was to blame for the crop of blisters that had sprouted on her tongue seemingly overnight. Her doctor thought otherwise. He had lost countless patients to AIDS in the last three years; with one look at Goldenberg's tongue, he told her she had AIDS. The lesions on her tongue weren't caused by hot coffee, he said; they were caused by oral thrush—a fungal infection that often results from a weakened immune system—and is a sign of AIDS.

Goldenberg refused to believe him. She thought he was "jumping on the [AIDS] bandwagon like every other doctor in town." Then three years later, just months before she planned to marry her boyfriend of four years, Goldenberg's soon-to-be mother-in-law casually mentioned that her son had "full blown AIDS." She asked Goldenberg, "Do you have it too?" Goldenberg went for a blood test and called off the wedding. Then she moved to Dallas.

Goldenberg recalls family members who stopped sharing plates and silverware with her after they heard the news. They warned her not to speak about her status. "My family said that was like washing dirty laundry in public," she says. But now she is a prolific public speaker and even an actress. At a conference in 2014, Goldenberg acted in a play about four women—two young and two old—who were diagnosed with HIV. "I didn't fit the picture of who I believed could get HIV. I thought my doctor didn't know what he was talking about," she said.

She said that even for her, an approachable woman with a broad smile, reaching out to other women with HIV—especially older women—can be difficult. "Some of these women are scared to meet me!" she exclaims. "We have to meet at McDonald's or someplace that is definitely not associated with HIV."

Finding safe spaces to share personal stories and establishing support networks is beneficial for both physical and emotional health. For older adults, good social support actually offers protection from sexually transmitted infections, according to Amin, the University of North Texas researcher.

But it can be difficult to find a place to connect with other older adults living with HIV. "There's not really anywhere else for them to go," said Melissa Grove, executive director of the Legacy Counseling Center in Dallas, a place that offers support to older adults, some of whom are living with sexually transmitted infections. Grove is organizer of the conference that Goldenberg takes part in most years. She said more than a third of the 200 or so HIV-positive women who attend the conference are aged 50 and older. The proportion of older women increases each year.

Besides tackling new medication regimens and the side effects that come with them, older adults diagnosed with HIV are dealing with the stigma that still surrounds the virus. "A lot of our clients are feeling fear, shame, and confusion," says Grove. "Usually, they haven't heard much about HIV/AIDS before their diagnosis, and they are so scared to tell anyone about what they're going through."

Seniors who were socially engaged—those who volunteered at local organizations or were involved with community groups—were less likely to have unprotected sex, compared with those who were less socially active, Amin found in his study. He says that's because socially engaged seniors have better access to sexual health information.

Staying active and informed helps older adults protect themselves from the increasing rates of sexually transmitted infections in their peer group. But the public health problem isn't that older people are having sex. It's that the rest of us are so shocked by it.

34

Did genetically modified mosquitoes spread Zika, and does the virus cause birth defects?

As the outbreak of Zika virus spread across the Americas starting in 2015, so did conspiracy theories about the virus. At the height of the epidemic, more than a third of Americans believed the Zika outbreak was caused by genetically modified mosquitoes, according to a survey by the University of Pennsylvania. The outbreak gained international attention, not because of the mild rash and aches and pains the virus caused, but because children born to mothers with Zika suffered birth defects such as shrunken brains and blindness. Scientists couldn't understand why a virus that usually caused a mild fever and headache was crossing the placenta and disabling, even killing, babies. The medical mystery fueled conspiracy theories about the little-known virus.

Zika was first discovered in 1947 by scientists studying yellow fever in Uganda's Zika forest. The word *zika* means "overgrown" in Luganda, one of the local languages. The scientists had trapped a monkey in a cage on a tree platform, and two days later the monkey was sick with a fever. The virus isolated from its blood was named after the forest, and the next year the same virus was discovered inside mosquitoes in the same area.

The virus and antibodies to it were first found in people in Uganda in 1952. In 1968, scientists also found Zika virus in the blood of people in Nigeria. As many as 40 percent of people in one part of Nigeria had Zika antibodies, meaning they had been infected with the virus at some point. The infection was discovered to cause a mild illness with rash, red eyes, and aching joints that lasted around five days. It's thought that eight out of ten people infected with Zika don't suffer any symptoms at all and for the rest, the illness might be mild enough that they may not seek medical attention.

Zika virus is spread by more than twenty species of mosquitoes, but most often by a kind called *Aedes aegypti* and *Aedes albopictus*. *Aedes aegypti* also spreads the dengue viruses, yellow fever, and chikungunya. The mosquitoes that spread these viruses are found in most parts of the world, although people who live in tropical and subtropical regions are most at risk.

By the 1980s, Zika had spread from east Africa to west Africa and to Asia, but only fourteen cases had been documented around the world. Then, the first major outbreak of Zika hit. It happened in 2007 in Yap, a small island in the Pacific Ocean in the Federated States of Micronesia. More than 100 people in Yap were probably infected with the virus for the first time.

"The emergence of Zika virus as an important human pathogen on Yap in 2007 underscores the ease with which exotic pathogens are transported between continents," the doctors working on the island who noticed the outbreak wrote in the *New England Journal of Medicine*. The virus likely spread from there to several Pacific islands. Starting in 2013, the biggest outbreak of Zika occurred in French Polynesia and spread to other Pacific islands including New Caledonia, the Cook Islands, and Easter Island.

But still not much attention was paid to the virus.

Until Zika virus arrived on the shores of Brazil. It was the virus's first foray into American waters. In August 2014, canoeists from around the world arrived in Rio de Janeiro for the Va'a World Sprint Championship canoe race. Among them were athletes from French Polynesia, New Caledonia, the Cook Islands, and Easter Island.

Four months later, residents of Pernambuco, a northeastern state in Brazil, were sick with Zika. By February and March, the states of Maranhao, Rio Grande do Norte, and Bahia were reporting cases.

But something was terrifyingly different. Besides the usual Zika symptoms of rash, aching joints, headaches, and red eyes, a new and horrifying symptom of Zika was emerging. Babies born to mothers infected with the virus suffered blindness and shrunken heads and brains. The birth defect, known as micro-cephaly, potentially linked to Zika was reported in twenty countries by 2016. That same year, the first Zika-related death in the United States was reported in a man in Utah.

If the virus had been circulating through Africa, Asia, and the Pacific Ocean for nearly seventy years, why hadn't it been linked to birth defects before? And how could a virus that usually caused a mild infection turn deadly?

The Brazilian outbreak, now the largest Zika epidemic in history, spread to more than a million people and is thought to have caused microcephaly in more than 4,000 babies. The vast majority of these cases were not proven to have been caused by Zika infection.

Immediately, theories about pesticides and biowarfare were debated. There was talk of bringing back a toxic, outlawed insecticide called DDT to kill Zi-ka-spreading mosquitoes.

But evidence soon mounted that Zika could cause birth defects. The virus was found in the amniotic fluid of pregnant women with Zika, and the virus was isolated from the brains of fetuses and babies with birth defects.

One way doctors can say a chemical or infectious disease causes harm to a fetus is by linking a rare chemical or bug to a rare birth defect. This rare exposure–rare defect approach was called "the astute clinician method" by Dr. Thomas Shepard, a pediatrician who spent much of his life working at the University of Washington.

The astute clinician method was the same approach used by Dr. Norman Gregg in 1941 to say maternal infection with rubella virus caused babies to be born with cataracts, a clouding of the lens in the eye. Gregg was an Australian ophthalmologist who pieced together the puzzle by noticing babies born with the eye condition had mothers who suffered infection with rubella early in their pregnancy. Gregg's discovery was made during a large outbreak of rubella in Australia that year. By talking to doctors around the country, he learned that they were seeing a similar thing and that the virus was causing other defects, including heart problems that killed many babies.

That same approach was used by doctors in 1973 to say that alcohol is a teratogen, the name given to something that causes harm to an embryo or fetus. In the case of alcohol, it causes a set of malformations known as fetal alcohol syndrome.

It was a bit of an ad hoc way to assess teratogens, and in the 1990s, Shepard was worried that there wasn't a framework that doctors could use when assessing whether something could be dangerous to a growing baby. He came up with "Shepard's criteria," a set of rules published in 1994 that can be used to figure out if something is a teratogen or not.

Shepard's criteria came in handy in 2015, when the spike in babies born with birth defects was reported in Brazil. Scientists used his seven criteria to ask if Zika virus was causing the malformations. Shepard's criteria included asking if the association makes biological sense. In this case it did. Zika was found to cause brain damage in animals, and it was found in the brains of babies born with defects. It also met the criteria for a rare exposure associated with a rare defect, plus, a very specific set of malformations was being seen. Shepard's criteria also asked for proof that fetuses had been exposed to the teratogen, a criterion that was met in the case of Brazil's outbreak, where pregnant women tested positive for the virus and later gave birth to malformed babies.

Shepard's list of seven criteria works in two ways. If the answer is yes to criteria 1, 3, and 4, then the exposure causes the birth defects because of the rare exposure–rare defect approach. But there's another way of looking at a potential teratogen and assessing if it really does cause harm to an unborn baby. It involves looking not at individual cases and trying to make a link but taking a step back and assessing the bigger picture. That means looking at epidemiologic trends and patterns and conducting case control studies. This approach is how it was discovered that the medicine valproate, which is used to treat epilepsy, causes the birth defect spina bifida if taken in the first trimester of pregnancy.

If the answer is yes to criteria 1, 2, and 3, the exposure causes the birth defect by the second approach, known as the epidemiologic method. In the case of Zika virus, it checked the boxes for criteria 1, 3, 4, and 6 and partially for criterion 2.

Then there was a new revelation. Brazilian babies were not the first to be born with birth defects because of Zika. Looking back at birth records during and after French Polynesia's Zika outbreak in 2014, researchers found at least seventeen babies were born with severe brain malformations, including microcephaly. The virus had caused birth defects before. No one had been paying attention.

Zika virus flourishes in the vagina and can spread to the uterus and cause damage to a fetus. Studies in 2016 found that the virus thrives in the vagina even in mice with robust immune systems. A study in humans found the virus can stay in the vagina for eleven days after infection. It was already known that as well as being spread through the bite of a mosquito, the virus can spread through unprotected sex. A man passed the infection to his partner through unprotected anal sex in Dallas in 2016.

There was also evidence that the virus was causing nerve damage in adults. Nearly 2,000 cases of Guillain-Barré syndrome were reported in Brazil by January 2016, mostly in states with outbreaks of Zika virus. Guillain-Barré syndrome is an illness caused by an immune system fired up over an infection, which then mistakenly attacks the lining of nerve cells.

A single amino acid substitution in the Zika virus shifted it from causing a mild illness to disfiguring babies' heads and brains. That was according to research by scientists at the Chinese Academy of Sciences who studied the virus in mice and compared old strains of Zika to the strain that recently had caused huge outbreaks. They injected strains of Zika that were circulating in 2015 and 2016 into the brains of day-old mice, and all the mice died. But when they injected mice with an old strain of Zika, fewer than a fifth of the mice died. When they did the same experiments with mouse embryos, the recent strains of Zika caused the embryos to develop microcephaly.

In the winter of 2018, Zika was actively circulating in more than eighty countries across Asia, Africa, the Pacific Islands, and the Americas. The Centers for Disease Control and Prevention was warning pregnant women to avoid these countries and advising anyone planning to get pregnant to wait three months after the male partner had returned from an area with Zika. That was because studies had shown the virus could linger in semen that long. If the woman had been to an area with Zika, she was advised to wait two months before trying to conceive.

At the height of the outbreak, governments of five countries told women to delay pregnancy for up to a year. In Brazil and Ecuador, women in areas hit hard by Zika were told to delay pregnancy indefinitely.

With proof that the virus did cause birth defects and that earlier instances of babies born with Zika-related malformations might have gone unnoticed, conspiracy theories about the mosquitoes that spread the virus persisted.

Was a mutant mosquito causing the world's biggest outbreak of Zika? Conspiracy theories often have a hint of truth, and in this case, scientists were tinkering with the genes of Zika-spreading mosquitoes. One approach to the epidemic was to set mosquitoes against mosquitoes. That might sound counterintuitive, but genetic modifications were used to make Zika mosquitoes less likely to pick up and spread the virus.

One of the many problems with the types of mosquitoes that usually spread Zika—unlike the kind that spreads West Nile virus—is that they like to stick really close to us and our homes. When trucks drive through the neighborhood spraying their fog of insecticide, the spray will hit the West Nile mosquitoes, which live closer to the street, but will probably miss the Zika mosquitoes closer to our homes.

That's why scientists were looking at genetic engineering as a tool instead of relying on chemicals. The other reason was because chemicals weren't working as well as they used to. Mosquitoes were becoming resistant to them. That had some people talking about bringing back a pesticide called DDT, which was banned in the United States in 1972. DDT was found to be toxic to the environment, but it was a very effective mosquito killer.

I visited a lab at the University of Maryland, where scientists were changing the immune systems of mosquitoes to make them resistant to viruses like Zika and dengue. The hope was that if these mosquitoes fed on the blood of a person infected with Zika or dengue, the mosquito wouldn't become infected.

Another idea was to infect the mosquitoes with a bacteria that limits the mosquitoes from spreading viruses. *Wolbachia pipientis* is a bacteria that infects many mosquitoes, but not the type that spread Zika. Scientists at the World Mosquito Program infected *Aedes aegypti* mosquitoes with *Wolbachia* and released them into the wild, where they mated with other mosquitoes and infected them. Over time, the scientists had to release fewer and fewer lab-infected mosquitoes because the ones they previously released had started a chain of infections throughout the mosquito population. The bacteria can also be used to make it harder for mosquitoes to reproduce.

A British firm called Oxitec was genetically engineering mosquitoes to make them suicidal. The company's CEO, Hadyn Parry, described it as "birth control for insects." Male mosquitoes made by Oxitec have a mutant gene that means their offspring can't reach adulthood. The mosquitoes die as babies. That means fewer mosquitoes and less spread of diseases such as Zika and dengue.

When his company first came to the United States, Parry said, "Who regulates mosquitoes?" and the response was, "We don't know." "It took us two years to find a regulator, and the [US Department of Agriculture] said mosquitoes are nothing to do with us," Parry said. "The FDA said it's not us. It's not a food and it's not a drug. So we kept going around in circles until finally the FDA said, 'We'll regulate it, and we'll set up a system where we bring in the CDC and the EPA and other institutions, and we'll be the coordinating agency.' It took us two years to find out who would be the lead agency." The technology was so new that there weren't systems in place to regulate it. Should these bugs be classified as insects or as a new kind of insecticide?

While it waited for US regulators to catch up with the pace of technology, Oxitec released its mosquitoes in Brazil. The company was churning out more than 30 million genetically modified mosquitoes every week in one of its Brazilian factories. Those mosquitoes were released by vans that let out small black clouds of bugs as they trundled down the streets of cities such as Piracicaba. Oxitec's transgenic bugs reduced mosquito populations by more than 90 percent, according to studies in Brazil and the Cayman Islands.

None of these mosquito-killing techniques are without risk. We don't know the long-term impact of releasing genetically engineered mosquitoes into the wild. If we wiped out *Aedes aegypti,* or reduced the mosquito population to much lower levels, what effect would that have on the animals that eat them and on the ecosystem as a whole?

But as mosquitoes spread across greater expanses of the world, so do viruses. From one corner of an African jungle in 1947 to seventy-two countries by 2007, the Zika virus was a fresh example of the craftiness of viruses and the human ingenuity needed to try and outrace them.

35

Can your cat's poop make you better at business?

An estimated 2 billion people around the world are infected with a brain parasite that some scientists say alters mood and behavior. Before you start blaming your erratic conduct on the bug, it's important to know that much of the research on *Toxoplasma gondii* has been done on mice, but a growing number of studies are looking at humans.

Toxoplasma gondii is a single-celled parasite found around the world. An estimated 40 to 60 million Americans are infected with the bug, mostly through eating contaminated and undercooked food, especially lamb, venison, and pork, or eating other foods contaminated by cooking utensils that had contact with undercooked meat. Water can also carry the parasite, and it can live in soil. The parasite can be spread from mother to child during pregnancy, and very rarely, the parasite is spread through organ donation.

Here's the cat connection. Despite the bug enjoying soil, water, organs, and meat, the only place that *Toxoplasma gondii* can reproduce is inside a cat's gut. So, while it can infect a range of animals, including mice and humans, the parasite really wants to get into a cat.

It does this by infecting mice and rats and changing their behavior. A rodent infected with *Toxoplasma gondii* develops a swagger that keeps it from running from a cat. It thinks the cat is its best friend. In some studies, rats infected with the parasite even become turned on by the scent of a cat.

Stupid mouse, you might say, but its bravery in the face of a feline foe is a cunning strategy of the parasite. By changing the behavior of an infected rodent, the parasite gives the cat a winning chance at pouncing and eating the animal. And the parasite ends up exactly where it wants to be: inside the cat's belly.

Infected cats shed millions of parasites in their poop for up to three weeks after they eat an infected mouse or other animal. If you accidentally touch your mouth after touching cat poop, you may ingest the parasite. This could happen after you clean out the litter box. *Toxoplasma gondii* is the reason doctors tell women to avoid changing cat litter during pregnancy.

The parasite infects many Americans every day, but people with a healthy immune system can usually fight off the infection. In pregnancy, however, the immune system is weaker; it's designed that way so the mother's body doesn't reject the fetus. In a pregnant woman or a person with a weakened immune system, the parasite establishes a full-on infection.

Most people infected with *Toxoplasma gondii* won't have any symptoms, others will feel like they have flu that lasts for a month. The parasite burrows into the brain and other organs and causes cysts throughout the body. In the eye, *Toxoplasma gondii* causes swelling and scarring that can lead to blindness.

Babies infected with the parasite can suffer brain damage and serious eye problems at birth, but most develop symptoms years later. These include mental disability and blindness.

So the parasite messes with the brains of rodents and changes their behavior. What does that have to do with your brain? A growing number of studies are linking *Toxoplasma gondii* to mental disorders in humans. In 2006, researchers found that people infected with the parasite were more likely to be neurotic.

In 2016, researchers at the University of Chicago found that people with a psychiatric disorder whose symptoms include explosive anger and road rage were twice as likely to have been exposed to the parasite.

That study was small; it included only 358 people. But in a larger study in Denmark looking at 45,000 children, scientists searched the children's blood for evidence that their mothers had been infected with the parasite. Then they looked at the mothers' medical history and found that women who had been infected with *Toxoplasma gondii* were 54 percent more likely to attempt suicide than uninfected women. Even women with no history of mental illness were more likely to harm themselves if they had been infected with the parasite.

Other studies have backed up the finding that in some populations, people who attempt suicide are more likely to have been infected with *Toxoplasma gondii*. Some studies have found that the risk of suicide is higher among infected patients who are also diagnosed with schizophrenia.

In analyzing 23 studies of more than 10,000 people, researchers found that those with schizophrenia were more likely to have antibodies to *Toxoplasma gondii*, meaning they had been exposed to the parasite at some point. Another study found that women with the parasite have babies who are at higher risk of developing schizophrenia.

But a 2016 study by researchers in New Zealand found the bug was not associated with changes in behavior. Scientists studied around 1,000 people; 28 percent tested positive for *Toxoplasma gondii*, but they were not more likely to have poor impulse control, criminal convictions, or signs of schizophrenia or depression. The one possible correlation was a higher risk of suicide attempts among people who tested positive for the parasite.

Scientists studying the mental health effects of *Toxoplasma gondii* turned their research question on its head in 2018. If the bug made humans engage in riskier behavior, could that be a good thing for people starting businesses? Most business ventures fail, meaning that successful entrepreneurs take big risks throughout their lives. Could people good at business be infected with the parasite?

In 2018, entrepreneurship researchers at the University of Colorado teamed up with biologists to study this question. They found that students with antibodies to *Toxoplasma gondii* in their blood were 1.4 times more likely to major in business studies and 1.7 times more likely to specialize in entrepreneurship, compared to those who had no evidence of previous infection to the parasite. Businesspeople attending entrepreneurship events were also included in the study. Those who tested positive for the bug were 1.8 times more likely to have started their own business venture.

The researchers looked at the prevalence of *Toxoplasma gondii* in forty-two countries over twenty-five years and combined these findings with data from the Global Entrepreneurship Monitor, which tracks entrepreneurial activity. Countries with a higher prevalence had higher "entrepreneurial activity and intentions at the national scale," the scientists said. Countries such as Brazil, which had a prevalence of 60 percent (compared to Norway, which had a prevalence of 9 percent), had a lower proportion of people who said fear of failure stopped them from starting new businesses.

While scientists aren't sure if the bug definitely impacts behavior, and if it does how that works, some believers of the hypothesis say it's a result of how our immune system handles the infection. It's humbling—and important—to think that a microscopic bug found in cat poop manipulates the behavior of mice and rats and might play a role in our mental health, too.

Indoor cats are less likely to harbor the bug, but if your cat hunts outside, wear gloves when gardening (since the cat might poop outside), cover children's sandboxes when not in use, and avoid cleaning the litter box when pregnant.

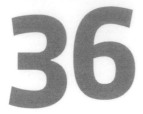

Is suicide contagious?

An outbreak of suicide was one of the first outbreaks I was asked to investigate when I joined the Epidemic Intelligence Service in 2011. My job was to track and stop epidemics. But I had expected to chase viruses, bacteria, and perhaps fungi across the States and around the world. Not an outbreak of suicide.

It turns out that it's not just microbes that are contagious; behaviors are contagious too. The outbreak of suicide was among Bhutanese refugees living in Arizona, Texas, Georgia, and New York.

Between 2008 and 2014, close to 80,000 refugees from Bhutan had settled in the United States, many of them had waited years, even a decade, to leave refugee camps and make a home in the United States. Bhutan, a small Himalayan nation renowned for having the world's highest "happiness index," was not a place associated with people who considered death by suicide. But the ethnic group settling in the United States was the Lhotsampas. They were descendants of Nepalese people who migrated to Bhutan in the late 1800s. But in the 1990s, they were forced to leave Bhutan and live in refugee camps in Nepal because of their ethnicity.

In 2012, the year after I joined the Epidemic Intelligence Service, the suicide rate among Bhutanese refugees in the United States was 24.4 for every 100,000 Bhutanese refugees—double the suicide rate for Americans.

The hardships of settling in an unfamiliar place, unemployment, poverty, dealing with the trauma of years living—even being born—in a refugee camp, the violence of being forced to leave home, were taking their toll.

One vital tool in suicide investigation is the psychological autopsy. Suicide is complicated, rarely driven by one thing and misunderstood because of the stigma surrounding mental illness. Psychological autopsies can help us understand what led a person to take his or her own life.

Psychological autopsies involve interviewing family members and friends of a person who died from suicide as well as talking to their doctors, if they were engaged in the health care system; and looking through medical notes. It brings together information from different people to paint a picture of the deceased person's life.

When investigators at the Centers for Disease Control and Prevention performed psychological autopsies to understand the clusters of suicides among Bhutanese refugees, they found that many people who had died from suicide had lived through the suicide of a family member or friend.

Can experiencing the suicide of a loved one, or even reading about the suicide of an unrelated person in the newspaper, influence a person's decision to take his or her own life?

In Goethe's novel *The Sorrows of Young Werther,* the young male protagonist takes his own life after a hopeless infatuation with Lotte, a fallout with his friend Albert (who is in a relationship with Lotte), and the death of his friend Hans. The book was published in 1774 and became very popular across Europe, catapulting Goethe from relative obscurity to literary stardom.

But soon after it was published, the novel was banned in Denmark, Italy, and Leipzig in Germany. Even Werther's style of clothing was forbidden. Two thousand young men took their lives in the same way as Werther, using a similar type of gun, wearing his style of clothing, it was reported. Many had the novel at the site of the suicide.

This was dubbed the Werther effect, the Young Werther effect, or Werther fever. Goethe's novel sparked a debate about the influence of Werther's story on young men and copycat suicides.

How to counter the contagion? The author Friedrich Nicolai wrote what would nowadays be called fanfiction. He penned a version of the story where Werther's friend Albert puts chicken blood in Werther's pistol and scuppers his suicide attempt. (This infuriated Goethe, who wrote a poem about Nicolai taking a dump on Werther's grave.)

The Werther effect is one of the earliest known examples of possible suicide contagion. Not everyone believes the phenomenon is real. In 1897, a century after *The Sorrows of Young Werther* was published, French sociologist Émile Durkheim wrote *Le Suicide,* a unique publication for its time, merging scientific methodology with suicide case studies. In *Le Suicide,* Durkheim writes that a person who dies from suicide would have died with or without experiencing the suicide of a loved one or hearing about another person's suicide.

The debate continues, and one example used by those arguing for the existence of suicide contagion is the story of the Vienna subway system. In 1983 there were no suicides and only one suicide attempt in the system. But in 1984, there were eight suicides and suicide attempts. That number increased to twenty-two in 1987.

Most involved men who were on average younger than those who died from suicide in Vienna outside of the subway system. Sometimes there were clusters of suicides, with up to five suicides a week at times; other times months passed with no suicides.

The Austrian press reported almost every single suicide since the increase beginning in 1984. Concerned about the impact of media reports and the potential for suicide contagion, researchers at the University of Vienna analyzed all reports of suicide printed in two of Austria's biggest newspapers.

They found journalists covering suicide wrote dramatic stories, and they discovered that suicides in the Vienna subway system dropped massively in the second half of 1987 right when guidelines for journalists covering suicide were released by the Austrian Association for Suicide Prevention.

"These media guidelines were based on the assumption that a certain kind of reporting on suicide may trigger suicidal behaviour," the researchers said. "The hypothesis was that reports on suicide may lead someone who is despairing to believe that committing suicide is the best and maybe only way out of his or her situation."

The researchers figured the "trigger effect" would be bigger when newspapers put the suicide story on the front page or included a photo of the person who had died. They said the imitation effect can be bigger when journalists covering suicide include too many details of the incident, say the person who died "had everything to live for," or report the motives as romantic, such as when a person chooses suicide to "join" a deceased loved one.

So the suicide prevention organization suggested that reporters include alternatives to suicide, such as sources of psychological support, and cover stories where a person at risk of suicide was helped and was able to overcome crisis.

This notion that suicide can be averted with the right support and that the media can play a positive role in preventing suicide contagion is called the Papageno effect after a Mozart opera that premiered in 1791, a few years after *The Sorrow of Young Werther* was published. *The Magic Flute,* an opera in two parts, tells the story of a bird catcher called Papageno, who tries to hang himself over a lost love but survives with the help of three spirits who remind him of his blessings.

Even though the Werther effect and the phenomenon of suicide contagion is still debated, it's considered best practice to follow the kinds of guidelines offered by the Austrian Association for Suicide Prevention. (In the United States, organizations such as Reporting on Suicide and others offer similar guidance to reporters.)

Their guidance is not always heeded.

In 2017, Netflix released a show about Hannah Baker, a fictional young woman, based on a young adult novel published a decade earlier. In twenty-six episodes *13 Reasons Why* tells Hannah's story after her death from suicide. Hannah leaves behind thirteen tapes detailing the thirteen reasons why she died. The tapes are found by Clay, a young man who had a crush on Hannah.

The show did all the things experts say you should not do when portraying suicide in fictional or nonfictional accounts: there was a scene showing the gory details of Hannah's death, and there was a scene portraying her death from suicide as a unifying event for her community.

In the nineteen days after the show was released, Google queries about suicide rose by almost 20 percent. That translated to 900,000 to 1.5 million more searches on suicide than usual, according to a 2018 study published in *JAMA Internal Medicine.*

An increase in internet searches about suicide doesn't mean there is an increase in suicides. But people were searching specifically for suicide methods, the scientists said. They added, "*13 Reasons Why,* in its present form, has both increased suicide awareness while unintentionally increasing suicidal ideation."

Dan Reidenberg is a suicide prevention expert and executive director of Suicide Awareness Voices of Education. He came to talk to my newsroom when I was a staff writer at the *Dallas Morning News.* He talked about how as reporters and editors we can influence behavior with our reporting and that journalism has the potential to raise awareness about mental illness, challenge stigma through storytelling, and shine a light on sources of support for people experiencing a crisis.

A month before *13 Reasons Why* was released, Netflix asked Dan to watch the show. Dan watched most of the episodes. Then he told Netflix not to release the show. "Although it's created a conversation about suicide, it's not the right conversation," he said to reporters. He said the show glamorizes suicide and sends harmful messages about seeking help, particularly in a scene where the high school counselor keeps answering his phone while Hannah is trying to get help. He even shifts blame for her feelings on to her.

"Young people are not that great at separating fiction from reality," he told the *Washington Post.* Dan and other suicide experts have suggested showing counseling as a tool that can actually help people through their mental health issues. Experts have also recommended deleting the death scene.

Suicide is the third leading cause of death among 15- to 19-year-olds in the United States, according to the CDC. In 2011, 16 percent of American high school students said they had seriously considered suicide. Clusters of teen suicides have been reported in places such as Palo Alto, California, and the towns of New Bedford and Needham in Massachusetts.

Teenagers are more vulnerable to suicide because their brains are developing, and the way the brain develops makes it difficult to process challenges and emotions. The parts of the brain that process emotion, including the amygdala, develop before the structures that regulate emotion. It's why sadness as a young person can feel especially overwhelming, sometimes insurmountable. (Remember your first romantic breakup?)

In teenaged brains or adult ones, the processes involved in suicide and suicidal ideation are complex. It's rarely one thing that leads a person to consider taking his or her own life, it's more often a constellation of factors, each of them tricky in its own right.

But as suicide survivors and experts will tell you, there is help, and psychological support can guide people safely through crises. If you or someone you know is in need of help, call the National Suicide Prevention Lifeline at 1-800-273-8255 if you are in the United States. A list of suicide support helplines from around the world are listed at http://www.suicide.org/international-suicide-hotlines.html.

37

Are suicide rates linked to the economy?

T wo years after Nancy Hobson's husband lost his job at Bank of America, he used a hunting gun taken from his family's vacation home to commit suicide. "The man and the job went together," said Hobson, who lives in Dallas, Texas. Her husband was "the life and center of every party," she said. But after he lost his job, "he really didn't know what to do having free time."

While many factors may have led her husband to take his life, several scientific studies point to a relationship between a bad economy and higher rates of suicide, especially among men.

Suicide rates have spiked during every recession since the Great Depression and have dropped during times of economic growth. During the economic crisis from 2008 to 2010, the suicide rate in the United States increased four times faster than it did during the previous eight years. The rate increased from about 11 suicides per 100,000 people to 12.5 per 100,000, according to researchers at the University of Cambridge in England.

There were 4,750 more deaths from suicide during 2008 to 2010, compared with the previous eight years. And for every rise of 1 percent in unemployment, there was a 1 percent increase in the suicide rate. The state with the strongest correlation between unemployment and suicide was Texas.

In the aftermath of the recession, Americans are more likely to die from suicide than from car accidents. And middle-aged adults—those most likely to lose their jobs during an economic crisis—have overtaken the elderly as the age group at highest risk of suicide.

A study by researchers at the Centers for Disease Control and Prevention looked at suicide rates from 1928 to 2007 and found that rates rose and fell with the economy. The suicide rate peaked in 1932, the last full year of the Great Depression, and fell to its lowest in 2000.

But sharp increases in unemployment, evictions, and home foreclosures after 2005 led to higher rates of suicide. Researchers at Rutgers University found that suicide rates rose with an increase in unemployment, and another group of CDC scientists found that suicides related to evictions and home foreclosures doubled from 2005 to 2010.

It's not always money worries that drive the unemployed to suicide. For men in particular, losing a job can mean losing their identity. Hobson's husband, Jack, was an investment banker who earned "about a million dollars a year" and was financially stable, she said. When he lost his job in 2010 after twenty-six years at the company, he received a generous severance package. The job loss didn't seem to have a financial impact on their lives.

"We were never big spenders to begin with," said Hobson. "After Jack lost his job we talked about cutting back . . . but we still ate at the same restaurants and he wasn't telling me, 'No you can't have that $30 entree off the menu.'" After losing his job, Jack stayed socially engaged, volunteering with his church and hosting dinner parties at their home.

Dawn Norris, assistant professor of sociology at the University of Wisconsin, La Crosse, said, "Our societal definition of masculinity is being employed, being the provider, being the breadwinner." She said that masculinity is linked to work, and without work, even wealthy men describe themselves as "impotent, deficient, worthless." Norris, an expert on job loss, gender, and suicide, interviewed hundreds of men with middle and upper-middle incomes who lost their jobs during the 2008 economic crisis.

"These are men who are financially secure, owned at least one home, had one or two cars," she said. "Their lifestyle was not really changing that much due to job loss." She asked them, "What does it mean to be a man?" They would say, "A man works. That's what a man is."

Americans work more than anyone in the developed world. Data from the Bureau of Labor Statistics show Americans now work longer, retire later, and take less vacation time than in previous decades.

With so much time spent at work, taking away a person's employment can mean not only taking away their identity but also the support network that would help them deal with the loss.

Le Suicide, the book by French sociologist Émile Durkheim published in 1897, argued that unemployment weakens our social integration and increases the risk of suicide. Durkheim proposed three theories for why this might be. In the "vulnerability" model, he explained that not having a job means having less access to support. In the "indirect causative" model, he said that unemployment leads to relationship and financial problems. In the "noncausal link" model, Durkheim proposed that a third factor means some people are at higher risk of both unemployment and suicide.

Suicide is hardly ever a result of one factor, said Benaye Rogers, chief philanthropy officer at St. Philip's School and Community Center, a faith-based organization in Dallas. Rogers is former president of Contact Crisis Line, an agency that provides telephone support to people who are feeling suicidal.

Rogers said that in early 2014 Crisis Contact Line experienced a 20 percent increase in calls from people contemplating suicide compared with the previous year. "When someone calls us, they usually have 10 things that are going on and affecting their mental health," she said. For "about 30 to 40 percent of people who are calling us, the underlying issue in their life is a result of the financial crisis."

Hobson says that her husband suffered depression, which was often precipitated by stress at work: "He would come home so often [during the economic crisis] and say, 'Today so-and-so was fired,' " she recalls. The severity of the depression peaked after he lost his job, but unlike the majority of men, Jack Hobson sought professional help and was given antidepressants.

The stigma surrounding mental health makes it difficult for many to get the support and medication they need. That's especially true for men, experts say. Men are less likely to speak openly about mental health issues, more likely to seek help later when problems are more established, and more likely to die from suicide than women.

More than 31,000 of the 39,518 Americans who died from suicide in 2011 were men. White men accounted for seven out of ten suicides in the United States in 2016, and overall, men are 3.53 times more likely to die by suicide compared to women, according to the American Foundation for Suicide Prevention.

That gender imbalance will lessen as women gain a firmer foothold in top-level jobs, say some suicide scholars. "Work at the moment isn't as central to who women are in society," says Norris. In one study, Norris found that women who lost their jobs during the economic crisis could shift from the role of breadwinner to another identity, such as mother, and better cope with unemployment.

The idea that job loss and economic downturn cause higher rates of suicide isn't new even if the data to prove that association is recent. "These new studies are not really saying anything new to those of us who work in the field of suicide every day," said Rogers.

Solutions to the trend include job creation and sustained economic growth—not always feasible, given the cyclical nature of the economy. Norris argues that a better work-family balance—as seen in some Scandinavian countries—will take the emphasis off work as the sole, defining feature in a person's life.

Providing support and helping people establish new social networks as they lose their jobs is another. "Those of us who have been able to rebound from depression have good family support," Rogers said. "We have good community support whether that's through our church or whether that's through neighbors."

Are there more suicides during the holiday season?

S ince religious institutions separated the body and the mind centuries ago, declaring the body the source of physical ailments and the brain the realm of the spiritual, mental illness has been stigmatized and misunderstood. Twelfth-century scholars dissected every part of the body below the neck but left the brain untouched.

We are still playing catch-up. "Pray it away," or "that person is weak, that's why they are depressed," are sentiments shared when talking about mental illness—if mental illness is talked about at all. One in four Americans experiences a diagnosable mental illness each year and yet, despite this being a shared human experience, the stigma persists.

Mental illness is not a personal failure. It can be a collective failure of society to support and care for people at the most vulnerable and difficult times in their lives.

Suicide rates in the United States have increased to their highest point in thirty years, according to the Center for Health Statistics. The rate increased

33 percent during 1999 to 2017. In 2016, close to 45,000 Americans died from suicide, compared with fewer than 30,000 in 1999. Suicide is now the tenth-leading cause of death across all ages and the fifth-leading cause among people 15 to 24.

Children are also at risk of suicide. Suicide rates among children 10 to 14 have doubled since 2007, according to the Centers for Disease Control and Prevention. Children in that age group are now more likely to die from suicide than in a car accident. In 2014, 425 children ages 10 to 14 died from suicide, compared with 384 who died in a car accident.

Not talking about these alarming trends or talking about them in alarmist ways can perpetuate falsehoods and stereotypes about mental illness. Vacuums of information breed taboos, which breed myths. That's especially true for suicide, considered a grave, unforgivable sin in some religions. The ideas that suicides increase in the holidays and that talking about suicides can trigger them are some of the myths that continue to spread. Some stereotypes, such as the notion of leaving a suicide note, are spread by television shows and movies.

Let's go through these one by one.

Suicide rates do not increase over the holidays, but it's a myth that is often perpetuated during the holiday season. The rate of suicide is actually lowest in December and there are more suicides during the spring. That trend is true for most of the Northern Hemisphere (the Southern Hemisphere sees a spike in suicides during its spring month of November). It's a trend that continues to puzzle mental health experts. Some attribute the increase to a hormone called melatonin, which is inhibited by sunlight. But that theory remains unproven.

There's even an academic institution that tracks the number of news stories about suicides spiking during the holidays. Over the 2009–10 holiday season, the Annenberg Public Policy Center at the University of Pennsylvania found that 50 percent of articles written during the holiday season perpetuated the myth. Things might be going in the right direction, however. In recent years there has also been an increase in news stories challenging the myth rather than supporting it.

Talking about suicide does not trigger suicide. In fact, the opposite can be true. If you're concerned that someone is considering suicide, it can be helpful to broach the subject with care. Talking about suicide does not increase a person's risk of dying from suicide. Language is important. Avoid words that stigmatize, including *commit,* which harks back to an age when suicide was considered a crime.

Most people who die by suicide do not leave a note. TV shows and movies often show characters leaving notes before they end their lives. It's a tidy way of wrapping up a story, but it's not true to life. In reality, about one in five who dies from suicide leaves a suicide note. For those who suffer the loss of a loved one to suicide, the expectation that there will be a note can add to their grief.

When there is a note, sometimes it's angry and blaming and it doesn't give closure the way the notes in the movies do, said Julie Cerel, a psychologist and professor at the University of Kentucky College of Social Work.

She looked through six years of suicide death data from Kentucky's national violent death reporting system to study any differences between people who leave a suicide note and those who don't. "I wanted to really dispel the myth that if there wasn't a note it couldn't be a suicide and to really help people whose loved one leaves a note or doesn't leave a note after they die by suicide. I wanted them to understand that very few people leave notes, it doesn't seem to be systematic in any way, and it doesn't really say anything about them."

She found that notes can be helpful and harmful and argued that TV shows should stop showing people writing suicide notes. "In the US pretty consistently, less than 20 percent of people that die by suicide leave a note. In our study it was like 18 percent. I think people have this great myth that the note would have helped me understand and feel at peace. But that never seems to happen."

Suicide is complicated and rarely caused by one thing. Instead, it's a combination of factors such as stress and mental health issues. If you are concerned about yourself or a loved one, there is help.

39

Are you more likely to die from a medical mistake than from a car crash?

When you place your life in a doctor's hands, you hope they will be diligent, competent, and caring. But according to one study, more Americans die at the hands of negligent doctors and nurses each year than from car crashes and respiratory diseases.

A quarter of a million Americans die each year because of medical errors, said researchers at Johns Hopkins University in a 2016 article published in the *British Medical Journal* (*BMJ*). That put medical mistakes as the third-leading cause of death in the United States, behind only heart disease and cancer. A documentary about medical mistakes released in 2018 said 440,000 people potentially died not in the hands of doctors but from the hands of doctors. The film, *To Err Is Human,* cited data from a 2013 study. The numbers were widely criticized as being overstated. That many deaths would imply that half of all people who die in a hospital die because of a medical error. Others said medical errors are underreported and these numbers might even be higher.

The study and the film generated scary headlines and may have put some people off seeing a doctor. But the researchers at Johns Hopkins who published the study on patient safety didn't visit hospitals or go through patient charts and death certificates. Instead they relied on data from four older studies and applied them to the number of people in hospitals in 2013 to estimate how many died from a medical error. It's not always a bad thing to pool data from older research, but it can cause problems, and in this case, the study was reported in the news as if the researchers had unearthed some new information about patient safety.

One of the four older studies the researchers looked at was a report from 1999 by the Institute of Medicine called "To Err Is Human." It's where the documentary film gets its name. In that report, it was estimated that between 44,000 and 98,000 Americans died each year from medical errors. The report was leaked to the press and had to be published before the official release date. News got out that a major network would feature a story about the report and the estimated 98,000 deaths from medical mistakes. The IOM said it hadn't wanted to scare patients or shame health care professionals. Its aim was to shine a light on health care systems, which can contribute to medical mistakes, and to look at ways to improve patient safety.

The data in *To Err Is Human* came from two other studies: one looking at patient safety in Utah and Colorado and another in New York. The study done in Utah and Colorado hospitals found that 6.6 percent of adverse events led to death and more than half of these adverse events happened because of a medical mistake that could have been prevented. In New York, the rate was higher. Nearly 14 percent of adverse events led to death and, again, half were due to medical mistakes.

It was the data from New York, which when extrapolated and applied to the whole of the United States, found that up to 98,000 Americans die each year because of medical errors. The Utah and Colorado study found 44,000 deaths could occur nationally each year from mistakes made in the hospital.

Medical mistakes are costly, the report said. It cited a study in two well-respected teaching hospitals where two of every hundred patients had an adverse event related to medications. The cost of these medication mistakes alone was $2.8 million a year for a 700-bed teaching hospital. The report again extrapolated this finding to the whole of the United States and said medication mistakes cost the country as much as $2 billion a year.

The second study that the Johns Hopkins researchers included in their analysis came from a study in ten North Carolina hospitals between 2002 and 2007. That study, published in 2010, was building on the 1999 report "To Err Is Human" and asked if efforts to improve patient safety had worked.

They hadn't. "We found that harm resulting from medical care was common, with little evidence that the rate of harm had decreased substantially over a 6-year period ending in December 2007," the authors of the North Carolina study wrote in the *New England Journal of Medicine*.

A third study included in the *BMJ* analysis was much larger and included 37 million Medicare discharges over a two-year period. Findings from that study were extrapolated and applied to the whole population of the United States. But there's the problem: Medicare recipients are 65 years or older, which can skew the data. For example, it's known that after surgery older people are more likely to suffer breathing problems than younger people and those breathing problems can lead to death.

A medical student at the University of Miami, Daniel Baldor, reanalyzed data included in the *BMJ* study and said the number of deaths from medical mistakes was 30.5 percent lower than the figure published by researchers at Johns Hopkins University. Baldor calculated an estimated 174,901 deaths from medical mistakes, which is a lot less than the quarter of a million previously calculated but still more than the annual number of deaths from car accidents and breast cancer combined.

But what constitutes a medical error? Some mistakes are clear cut. "The knowledgeable health reporter for the *Boston Globe*, Betsy Lehman, died from an overdose during chemotherapy. Willie King had the wrong leg amputated. Ben Kolb was 8 years old when he died during 'minor' surgery due to a drug mix-up." So starts the IOM's report on medical mistakes.

One challenge with all of the studies is the way they define a medical mistake. In medical school, we're taught that errors can happen during diagnosis (using the wrong test, coming up with the wrong diagnosis, taking too long to figure out why a person is sick); during treatment (a nicked blood vessel in the operating room, giving the wrong dose of medicine); or simply by having a poor bedside manner and being a terrible communicator.

In the *BMJ* article, the researchers say a medical error is any action "that does not achieve its intended outcome" or any planned action that if not done "may or may not cause harm to the patient."

But that broad definition doesn't differentiate between the doctor who prescribed double the dose of a medicine, the one who nicked an artery during a technically difficult surgery, or the one treating a patient with multiple, serious conditions. (And let's be honest, there are doctors who refuse to take in patients with multiple, complicated medical conditions because they don't want their death to skew their mortality data.)

The broad definition also doesn't take into account that the cause of death is sometimes impossible to determine. That means the information that ends up on the death certificate—the information often used in studies like the one we're talking about—is misleading.

Death certificates are themselves a problem. There is no diagnostic code for death from medical error. That leaves researchers with the difficult job of figuring out if death from kidney failure means a person's kidneys shut down because of a disease or if a medical mistake contributed to the fatal illness.

The point of talking about medical mistakes is not to scare patients away from hospitals and clinics but to address a very human, and often systemic, problem and come up with the solutions.

One set of solutions comes from the airline industry, which is often touted to doctors as one of the most risk-averse industries and one that patient safety can be modeled on. It's an industry that uses checklists, works to get rid of hierarchies so that junior staff feel empowered to speak up to seniors if they see a problem, and promotes a culture of safety. Medicine is often fiercely hierarchical and has a culture of blame, which doesn't help when it comes to learning from mistakes.

Many medical mistakes arise from flaws in the system. One example is electronic medical records, which were meant to make things safer and simpler, but can take time away from direct patient care and make things feel more complicated.

Some mistakes are a combination of human error and imperfect systems that are supposed to be our fail-safes. I remember an elderly patient of mine who had survived the Auschwitz concentration camp and nearly died in my hospital after I left for the night. The woman was allergic to penicillin but was given penicillin for an infection. This occurred despite the fact that I had followed protocol, put a red band on her wrist that said she was allergic, and documented her allergy in the paper medical notes and in the electronic medical record. Shouldn't the system have blocked a prescription of penicillin from ever being written for her in the first place? Shouldn't it have flagged the error to a person in the pharmacy department? Shouldn't it have prompted a nurse to see a red flag in the computer system at the time of administering the medicine, even if the nurse missed the red wristband?

There will never be an acceptable number of deaths or people harmed from medical mistakes—unless that number is zero. What's especially concerning about studies like the one published in the *BMJ* and documentaries such as *To Err Is Human,* is the scary headlines they generate and that they can prevent people from going to see a doctor. The health care system, flawed as it is, saves many more lives than it harms. Late diagnosis of many illnesses, including heart disease and cancer, can be deadly.

40

Is it dangerous to go to the hospital in July?

Medical lore says don't get sick in the summer. That's when new doctors, fresh out of medical school, are let loose on the wards and residents take on jobs with more responsibility.

It's not just medical myth. More than 300 studies have looked into this phenomenon and some show that your chance of dying in a hospital increases in July. To get to the bottom of this, researchers at the University of California, San Francisco (UCSF), sifted through thirty-nine studies conducted between 1989 and 2010. They looked at how patients fared in hospitals in July compared with other months.

They concluded: "Mortality increases and efficiency decreases in hospitals because of year-end changeovers." Some of the studies they looked at found a 4 percent increase in deaths during July. Others noted a 12 percent increase. Some found no difference in death rates in July.

The studies they looked at spanned more than two decades. There were a lot of changes to the medical system during that time, including the 2003 law that restricted the number of hours trainee doctors were allowed to work. Studies of the impact of that change say the 2003 duty-hour restrictions were associated with reductions in the number of deaths from heart failure, stroke, and pneumonia.

A study the UCSF researchers didn't look at found that the death rate in July went up but only for very sick patients. Researchers at Harvard Medical School studied about 75,000 heart attack patients who were admitted to hospitals during May and July. They separated the patients into two groups: those at high risk of dying from the heart attack (because of their age and other medical problems) and those at low risk of dying.

The Harvard researchers were careful to also separate hospitals into two groups, something that many other researchers overlooked. They put teaching hospitals in one group and defined them as places where a lot of patient care is delivered by resident physicians, meaning doctors in training. In the other group they put nonteaching hospitals, where patients are cared for by more experienced doctors.

Here's what they found: If you are a high-risk patient, then your chance of dying in a teaching hospital is lower than in a nonteaching hospital for most of the year.

Except in July. In July, high-risk patients in teaching hospitals faced the same risk of death as patients in nonteaching hospitals.

To give you an idea of the numbers, the chance of death for high-risk patients in a teaching hospital was 20 percent in May. In July, that went up to 25 percent—the same chance of death as in a nonteaching hospital.

For the low-risk group (those who had a heart attack but had a slim chance of dying because of their age and other factors), there was no July effect. So why were the high-risk patients more likely to die in hospitals in July compared with May? One explanation is that new trainees simply lack the experience of fully trained doctors. Some researchers say it's less about experience and more to do with a new doctor's lack of familiarity with a new hospital and its systems.

In a study of pediatricians at Children's National Health System, a teaching hospital in Washington, DC, there was a spike in medical errors by trainee pediatricians in July and far fewer mistakes in August. But there was not an increase in adverse patient events during July.

"The reasons for this were not explored in this initiative; however, we postulate that the hospital had more reported medical errors in July due to mistakes by the influx of new doctors and increased responsibility of trainees promoted to the next level of training," the authors wrote.

They also saw an increase in medical mistakes made by trainee doctors in September. Although they couldn't explain why, they wondered if by September the new doctors had more autonomy and were making difficult decisions on their own. Perhaps there's a September effect?

An increase in errors and a drop in efficiency during a big staff turnover isn't seen only in medicine. It's true of other industries as well. Studies have shown that employee turnover is bad for an organization's efficiency, whether that organization employs craftsmen, psychologists, or dieticians.

So, should you postpone that surgery you have scheduled in July? Probably not. Hospitals have systems in place to catch medical errors. In case the July effect is real, some hospitals have added measures in place to mitigate that effect. That can include more training for new doctors as well as better supervision systems. They're not foolproof by any means, but your chance of dying in a hospital isn't generally higher in July than the rest of the year. For hospitals adding safeguards in case the July effect is real, July could be the safest time to go to a hospital.

The July effect really refers to a patient's perception of mistakes made by medical professionals as an influx of fresh faces floods the hospital. It's about a patient's experience of medical care. While it's normal to be nervous during any hospital stay, it's expected that a patient might be more anxious when faced with doctors unfamiliar with their surroundings and their new accolade. (As a new doctor I would encourage my patients to call me by my first name. It took me some time to get used to being called "doctor.")

While anyone might be nervous (including the new doctors), the July effect seems to mostly affect those patients who have a high risk of dying from their illness in the first place. And their risk of death, according to some studies, was the same whether they were treated by newly qualified doctors or very experienced ones. More research into the July effect is helping hospitals make staff changeover and new employee induction safer and less frightening for patients and their health care teams.

41

Do patients cared for by female doctors live longer?

Men are more likely to survive a heart attack, and women are more likely to die. Women suffer different heart attack symptoms from men, things like pain in the neck, stomach, and jaw, a general sense of feeling unwell, pressure in the chest. These symptoms are more likely to be dismissed by doctors and the women themselves as indigestion or stress. Women are less likely to get to a hospital early, and even when they do go to a hospital, women are still more likely to die of a heart attack compared to men.

In 2018, researchers at Cornell University wondered if a woman's dire prospects could be explained or even made worse if she was treated by a male doctor. To answer that question they looked through the records of more than half a million patients treated for a heart attack in Florida hospitals between 1991 and 2010. Their findings confirmed what some doctors had been saying all along.

Not only did female patients fare better when they were treated by a female doctor, but *all* patients fared better if they were looked after by a female doctor. This survival effect was strongest for female patients.

The study by Cornell researchers was published in 2018, but it was hot on the heels of other studies looking at the same phenomenon. In a study published in the *Journal of the American Medical Association* in 2017, scientists at Harvard found elderly patients cared for by female doctors live longer and are less likely to return to the hospital than if they are cared for by a man. They calculated that 32,000 Americans would be saved each year if "male physicians could achieve the same outcomes as female physicians."

The researchers looked at more than 1.5 million Medicare patients hospitalized at some point during January 2011 to December 2014. Patients who were cared for by female doctors had a lower death rate—11.07 percent compared with 11.49 percent for patients with a male doctor—and lower readmission rates—15.02 percent compared with 15.57 percent. While those differences might seem small, the authors compared them to the overall reduction in death for Medicare patients over a decade, a reduction that was heralded as a major improvement.

The study compared doctors within the same hospital and found that patients with female doctors did better even when taking into account patients who were severely sick and comparing patients with different illnesses.

In a Canadian study looking specifically at surgeons, patients treated by female surgeons were less likely to die within thirty days, be readmitted, or suffer complications within thirty days. The study included more than 104,000 patients.

Earlier studies showed that men and women practice medicine differently. The differences begin in medical school, where women outperform men in medical school exams.

Once qualified and on the ward, female doctors are more likely to practice what's known as evidence-based medicine and to follow clinical guidelines. They're also less likely to treat patients differently depending on the patient's sex. A 2009 study analyzing how heart failure patients were treated showed that male doctors favored male patients in the way they prescribed medicines. The study also found that female doctors provided more thorough drug treatment to patients according to protocols.

Female doctors provide care that's centered around a patient's desires, other studies have shown. Women value their patients' needs and opinions and make them feel empowered so that they ask questions and share their perspective, according to a 2002 study focusing on physician communication. Female doctors are more likely to talk to a patient about the patient's home and work situation.

Female doctors are also more likely to order screening tests such as mammograms and Pap smears for their patients. These tests are designed to detect illnesses before they cause significant harm.

In a study from 1993, researchers at the University of Rochester found patients with female doctors were more likely to have screening for breast and cervical cancer, although no difference was found in the rate of screening for high blood pressure.

Outside of the hospital, Canadian researchers found, having a female primary care doctor means you are less likely to wind up in the emergency room. They studied the patients of 4,195 primary care doctors and found that, as well as doing a better job at cancer screening and managing diabetes, patients of female doctors were at lower risk of an emergency room visit or a hospital admission.

The authors concluded that "the indicators assessed in this study point to a benefit for patients under the care of female physicians." They suggested the difference could be a result of more referrals to specialists by female primary care doctors as well as a more patient-centered approach to medicine.

Despite providing better patient outcomes, female doctors earn around $20,000 less per year in the United States than their male counterparts. In a study of twenty-four medical schools in twelve states, researchers found that female doctors earn 8 percent less than male doctors.

In some cases, it's even harder to get into medical school as a woman. In 2018, one of Japan's most prestigious medical schools admitted to fudging women's entrance exam scores so that they appeared lower. The medical school wanted to limit the number of women who qualified to become doctors.

Once women pass that hurdle, there's the challenge of earning a fair wage. Analyses of scientist salaries show that women are offered substantially smaller faculty start-up packages. Male faculty were offered a funding package that was 67.5 percent higher than the sum offered to women faculty members, according to a study published in the *Journal of the American Medical Association* in 2016.

And even reaching the rank of full professor is more challenging for women. Male doctors are more than twice as likely as female doctors to reach the status of full professor.

Understanding exactly how female doctors provide superior medical care (despite taking home less money) could help all doctors improve their patients' outcomes. If you're thinking of rushing to switch to a female doctor, the good news is that at least half of medical school students in the United States are women. The bad news is that only one in three practicing doctors are female. That's because obstacles such as lower salaries and discrimination in academia mean women miss out on fulfilling careers—and patients miss out on the best clinical care.

42

Can a pill make racists less racist?

The actress Roseanne Barr blamed the medicine Ambien for her racism in 2018, when she tweeted that Valerie Jarrett, a Black woman who was advisor to President Barack Obama, looked like an ape. Ambien, a sedative used to treat insomnia, does not cause racism. The drug company that makes Ambien responded as such, saying: "While all pharmaceutical treatments have side effects, racism is not a known side effect of any Sanofi medication."

But Barr wasn't the first person to link racism to medication. In 2012, psychologists at Oxford University said a drug used to treat heart disease made people *less* racist. The study incited headlines around the world. Could a medicine taken by millions of people really be used to treat heart palpitations and racism?

The Oxford experiment was a very small study of thirty-six people, half of whom were given 40 milligrams of the medicine propranolol, which is from the class of drugs known as beta blockers. Beta blockers make the heart beat more slowly and with less force. The drug also lowers blood pressure and, as well as treating heart disease, it's used to treat anxiety and panic disorders.

All of the participants in the Oxford study were white Brits or Americans. After taking either the medicine or a placebo, they were asked to take a test called the implicit association test, or IAT, which detects and measures implicit biases. Those are the stereotypes and attitudes we hold that affect our decisions and behaviors in an unconscious way. The scientists who invented the IAT in the late 1990s said memories we are unaware of influence attitudes, and the IAT was designed to measure these unconscious thoughts.

The Oxford study was based on earlier findings from at least four experiments in the early 2000s that found increased brain activity in white people when they were shown photos of Black people. In particular, a part of the brain called the amygdala was activated in the white participants. The amygdala is an almond-shaped piece of gray matter that sits deep in the temporal lobe. It's the main part of the brain involved with emotions such as fear, arousal, and anger and is responsible in part for the fight or flight response. These earlier studies found links between the amount of amygdala activity in a person's brain and their IAT score. A study in 2000 found that increased activity in the amygdala was associated with implicit bias.

Propranolol has an effect on the amygdala. The drug works by blocking the activity of a chemical called norepinephrine, which is made by the adrenal glands on top of the kidneys. Norepinephrine is both a hormone and a nerve transmitter. It's one of the two main stress hormones in the body, along with cortisol.

Norepinephrine is responsible for making your heart race and your airways open. It also increases your blood sugar—all things necessary in the fight or flight response. In experiments, blocking the effects of norepinephrine with propranolol made people have less of an emotional response to stimuli and made their blood pressure go down in situations where it might be expected to go up. The opposite happened when people were given a drug that amplified the effects of norepinephrine. Those people became more angry or aroused when presented with stimuli, and their blood pressure and heart rate increased.

Norepinephrine also plays a role in our emotional memory. It is crucial in the process in which our memories are laid down and maintained, and it works in and with the amygdala to do this. Those memories you have of your childhood dog dying, your first kiss, or your baby being born are especially vivid and long-lasting because of norepinephrine. You're unlikely to forget those events, compared to a day of work, grocery shopping, and the gym. Those are considered emotionally neutral events, and norepinephrine won't be as engaged in laying down memories about them.

If you block the action of norepinephrine using a drug like propranolol, the level of activity in the amygdala is reduced and emotional memories are less likely to be created, maintained, and recalled.

The Oxford scientists wondered if emotional responses that are influenced by norepinephrine play a role in implicit bias. "The amygdala plays a key role in the early non-conscious appraisal of threat, and may therefore also be involved in the mediation of implicit racial prejudice," they wrote. So they took their group of thirty-six white people, gave half of them one dose of propranolol and the other half a placebo, and had them take a test for explicit bias and then a test for implicit bias.

In the explicit bias test, they were asked to score their feelings about different groups of people such as Muslims, gay people, white people, and Black people on a scale of zero to 100. The implicit bias test was a computerized test of negative and positive words that appeared on the screen with pictures of faces of Black and white people. Participants had to sort through the images as quickly as possible leaving little time for thinking. Their level of prejudice was calculated according to differences in the time they took to sort through blocks of negative and positive words.

Here's what happened.

Propranolol did not have any effect on their explicit biases. But the drug significantly reduced implicit bias as measured by the computer test. This could have happened because propranolol lowers the heart rate and blood pressure and these bodily effects are the ones that trigger negative implicit attitudes, the researchers speculated. Or, propranolol was interfering with amygdala activation, and that part of the brain really is central to implicit bias.

The authors said this was evidence that racism is founded on fear. One of the scientists involved with the study, Julian Savulescu, a professor in Oxford's philosophy department, told reporters: "Such research raises the tantalizing possibility that our unconscious racial attitudes could be modulated using drugs, a possibility that requires careful ethical analysis."

He was quick to point out that propranolol was not a treatment for racism. "Biological research aiming to make people morally better has a dark history. And propranolol is not a pill to cure racism. But given that many people are already using drugs like propranolol which have 'moral' side effects, we at least need to better understand what these effects are."

Other researchers are looking at different hormones and even brain stimulation as ways to fight racism. The year before the Oxford study was published, researchers in the Netherlands published a study about the hormone oxytocin. It's the chemical sometimes referred to as the "love hormone," but in the Dutch study, oxytocin was found to increase favoritism toward people like us, not people who are different. Dutch men in the study were shown six people and told they could only pick five they had to save on a lifeboat with limited space. The men who had been given oxytocin were more likely to reject men with Muslim and non-Dutch sounding names and more likely to save men with Dutch names. Whereas men who were given placebo didn't seem to pay attention to religion or ethnic origin when it came to saving lives.

These studies add to a body of research that shifts racism from a social problem to a medical one. One that can be medicated away. Except it's not an easy fix. And in a society where explicit bias, not just implicit bias, is still a life-threatening problem, focusing on implicit bias can feel like a cop-out since, well, we all have implicit biases and they're based on thoughts and memories that are unconscious and therefore uncontrollable.

The medicalization of racism strips it of its violent history, a history in which race was created as a social construct to dominate people deemed inferior because of supposed biological differences. Shifting the focus back to biology and adding in modern day medicine frames racist people as victims of a cerebral pathology. A pill can't cure racism because racism isn't a medical phenomenon.

43

Are airplane condensation trails, aka chemtrails, bad for your health?

Scientists call them contrails. Conspiracy theorists call them chemtrails. Whatever you call them, the white streams of condensation made by plane engines streak the sky and cause controversy.

In an international survey by researchers at Harvard and the University of Calgary in 2011, about 3 percent of people said it was "completely true" that a secret government program uses planes to spray dangerous chemicals into the air, and one in six believe this claim is at least partly true.

Conspiracy theorists say chemtrails linger in the air because they contain aluminum, strontium, and barium and that these chemicals are used to control humans, pollute food and water supplies, and change the weather. Scientists argue that contrails, short for condensation trails, are made when hot exhaust from a jet engine condenses in the cold, thin air at high altitude. The exhaust contains carbon dioxide, nitrogen oxide, sulfur dioxide, as well as soot, unburned fuel, and water vapor, which forms ice crystals. Aluminum, strontium, and barium that chemtrail conspiracy theorists claim are in the trails are naturally occurring in the earth's crust, scientists say, and that's why they show up in the soil samples some believe are contaminated.

Back in 2000, a group of US science agencies including the National Aeronautics and Space Administration, Environmental Protection Agency, Federal Aviation Administration, and National Oceanic and Atmospheric Administration published a fact sheet about contrails.

They explained that contrails are formed by a mixture of water vapor from a plane's exhaust fumes and the low temperatures in the atmosphere when planes cruise a few miles above earth. The white streaks in the sky are mostly ice crystals and are not harmful to humans, they said.

The first peer-reviewed study about condensation trails was published in 2016. "Quantifying expert consensus against the existence of a secret, large-scale atmospheric spraying program" was written by researchers at Stanford University and the University of California, Irvine.

SLAP. That's the acronym for the supposed Secret, Large-scale Atmospheric spraying Program government conspiracy they were talking about. The researchers asked seventy-seven geochemists and experts in atmospheric science about chemtrails and whether there is any evidence to support a SLAP. Seventy-six of the seventy-seven said that there was no evidence of a SLAP and that what conspiracy theorists point to as proof can be explained by chemicals naturally found in the atmosphere and by the physics of airplane emissions.

Airplanes rushing through the sky create pockets of high air pressure beneath them and low air pressure above. In the areas of low pressure, air cools and forms clouds. The water that cools can condense on the particles left behind by the aircraft, that mix of unburned fuel and soot.

Contrails are staying in the air longer, a third of the experts said. Bigger planes with bigger engines and aircraft flying at higher altitudes to allow for more planes to share the sky were some of the reasons why.

The one scientist who said there might be evidence of a SLAP cited evidence of "high levels of atm[ospheric] barium in a remote area" that usually had low levels of barium in its soil.

Scientists have tried to debunk the chemtrail conspiracy theory before—but not very often. In this new paper, the researchers say there haven't been enough attempts to dispel myths about military and government conspiracies and chemtrails. That raises the quandary about whether debunking conspiracies gives them legitimacy and extends their reach (more on that in the final chapter).

In this case, the scientists conducting the first peer-reviewed study on condensation trails said their "goal is not to sway those already convinced that there is a secret, large-scale spraying program—who often reject counter-evidence as further proof of their theories—but rather to establish a source of objective science that can inform public discourse."

Conspiracy theories about chemtrails are said to have picked up with the advent of the internet. There are a huge number of websites dedicated to the chemtrails conspiracy theory. What complicates things is that sometimes planes do spray chemicals that mess with the weather. It's called climate geoengineering, and it is a technique used to make clouds form rain. In cloud seeding, scientists spray dry ice and silver iodide onto clouds to make rain. It's been used in the Middle East and in California, where officials at the California Department of Water Resources said geoengineering increased rainfall by 4 percent a year.

If you think chemtrails are part of a government- or military-operated SLAP, you're not alone. A bunch of celebs endorse the chemtrail theory including Erykah Badu, Kylie Jenner, Billy Corgan of the Smashing Pumpkins, and Beck, who wrote a song about chemtrails. *I can't believe what we've seen outside, you and me watching the jets go by . . . All I can take from these skies is fog, and all I can see in this light . . . That's what I mean when we talk in this jet stream, we're climbing a hole in the sky.*

Some hard-line conspiracy theorists have threatened violence against scientists who try to debunk the myth. In his book, *A Case for Climate Engineering,* Harvard scientist David Keith describes how scientists who debunk SLAP and study geoengineering have been threatened by those who say the conspiracy theories are real. Keith is a professor of applied physics and public policy at Harvard University who has enraged climate activists by suggesting that a sun filter could be created to protect us from global warming. Keith has received death threats.

But now the experts have spoken, and they are pretty much in consensus. The trails left by plane engines are simply ice crystals condensed with hydrocarbons and the spill of jet exhaust. The government is not trying to kill us through the clouds, although that's not to say that government programs haven't maimed people before. But in the case of chemtrails, consider this conspiracy theory debunked.

44

Do bad teeth cause heart disease?

P eople with unhealthy mouths were up to three times more likely to suffer strokes and 50 percent more likely to suffer heart attacks according to studies by scientists in the United States and Sweden. Nearly half of all heart attack patients in the Swedish study had gum disease.

In the hopes of getting us to brush and floss better, dentists warn patients that oral health is linked to heart health, but what do your teeth have to do with your heart? When doctors and dentists say the state of your mouth impacts the health of your heart, they're really talking about gum health. There are two main types of gum disease. Gingivitis, where the gums are sore, swollen, red, and possibly receding and bleeding can occur when you brush your teeth or floss. Periodontitis is more serious. It happens when pockets form around the teeth and swollen gum tissue pulls away from the teeth. Teeth can eventually loosen and fall out.

Between one-third to one-half of Americans have some form of periodontitis, according to the Centers for Disease Control and Prevention. Almost one in ten suffer with a severe form of the disease, according to a 2012 survey. But don't rely on warning symptoms to alert you to the fact that you have gum disease. Many people with mild to moderate gum disease don't suffer any symptoms at all.

Gum disease, heart disease, and stroke share a common pathological theme: inflammation. Heart attacks and a type of stroke called ischemic stroke are caused by fat building up in the arteries that feed the heart and brain. But while we focus often on the fat that narrows these arteries, there's a lot more going on in the blockages than just fat.

When fat deposits inside blood vessels, it sparks an inflammatory process. White blood cells are lured to the scene, and calcium and platelets get involved, too. Calcified plaques are brimming with these cells and deposits. They narrow and stiffen the blood vessels and starve tissues of vital oxygen and nutrients.

In a Swedish study published in 2016, scientists examined the gum health of more than 1,600 people, including 805 people who had suffered heart attacks and 805 people who had no history of heart disease. Studying oral x-rays of the participants, they found a third had at least mild periodontitis. But when they compared the two groups, they found people with gum disease were almost 50 percent more likely to have a heart attack, compared to those with healthy gums.

Another thing that gum disease and heart disease have in common is bacteria. Gums are very vascular, and gum disease means you are more likely to bleed while brushing and flossing. When this happens, bacteria from the mouth enter the bloodstream and even enter the fatty plaques narrowing arteries. This fuels more inflammation within the blood vessels and can even contribute to an infection within the heart itself. Cutting open a plaque blocking a vessel, scientists have discovered a range of oral bacteria inside.

That's why people who are at risk of a heart infection called infective endocarditis are told to take antibiotics before having dental work done. The antibiotics prime the bloodstream with chemicals that can attack the bacteria before it settles in the heart.

In a study published in 2015 in the *Journal of Dental Research*, researchers studied 112 people who suffered a heart attack. They found that periodontitis was a risk factor for death from heart attacks.

231

Those findings back up recommendations published jointly by the *Journal of Periodontology* and the *American Journal of Cardiology* in 2009. In that report, the authors wrote that gum disease is a risk factor for heart disease and strokes. Analysis of data from a large, national dataset, the National Health and Nutrition Examination Survey, also highlighted gum disease as a risk factor for heart disease and strokes.

But when the American Heart Association reviewed hundreds of studies on gum disease and heart health, it found that, overall, there wasn't sufficient evidence to say that gum disease caused strokes and heart attacks. In 2012, a committee of the AHA looked at 537 studies investigating gum disease, fatty buildup in the arteries, stroke, and heart attack. While some studies showed an association between oral health, strokes, and heart attacks, the AHA said many studies showed no correlation. The authors of the study concluded that they couldn't say for certain that treating gum disease would definitely prevent heart disease. "Observational studies to date support an association between periodontal disease and atherosclerotic vascular disease independent of known confounders. They do not, however, support a causative relationship."

The link between gum disease and heart disease could simply be that the two share common risk factors. For example, rates of periodontitis are highest among people who smoke, have diabetes, and are obese. Those are the same risk factors for stroke and heart disease.

Or the link could be explained by the fact that people who neglect their teeth and gums by not brushing and flossing regularly are also less likely to exercise, eat a healthy diet, or visit the doctor regularly—all of which are essential for a healthy heart.

While dentists and cardiologists alike continue to debate the link between gum disease and heart disease, a report published in the *Journal of Periodontology* and the *American Journal of Cardiology* recommends that people with heart disease and any signs of gum disease talk to a dentist and that anyone with moderate to severe gum disease and a risk factor for heart disease, such as diabetes, should see a doctor. Dentists play a role, too. They are advised to tell patients with severe gum disease that they are at an increased risk for heart disease and strokes.

45

Can your zip code predict when you will die?

I n the 900 block of Brentwood Road in northeast Washington, DC, two and
a half miles from where I am writing this chapter, the average life expectancy
is 73 years and 1 month. If you live four miles away, on Kalorama Circle in
northwest DC, you can expect to live more than ten years longer. The average
life expectancy there is close to 81 years.

Your zip code determines how much you will earn, how sick you will get, and
when you will die. The average life expectancy in the United States is 81.1 years
for women and 76.1 years for men, but these averages vary wildly depending
on where we live. The difference of a few blocks is the difference between living
into your eighties or dying in your early seventies.

"If DNA is our biological blueprint, ZNA (zip code at birth) is the blueprint
for behavioral & psycho-social makeup," said Dr. Francis Collins, director of
the US National Institutes of Health, in a 2015 tweet.

That means before children enroll in school, before they even learn to hold
a spoon or a pencil, we can predict how much of a life those children will live.

It depends on which neighborhoods they call home.

More than our genes, our environment determines our wellness—and our sickness. We used to think individual behaviors played the biggest role in a person's health. Doctors would even blame patients (some still do) for developing type 2 diabetes or lung disease because of the foods they ate or their addiction to cigarettes. Now we understand that while personal choices and behaviors play a role in health, the biggest factors in determining health are those that usually can't be controlled by a person: things like what class you were born into, the color of your skin, how easy it is for you to get a steady job.

Then there's this lede from the news site NewsOne.com, which describes how neighborhoods where Black and brown people live have been targeted by some companies. "Leslie Adamson said the white truck that stopped at the Boston housing project she grew up in brought adults and children running, much like a visit from the ice cream man. But instead of sweets, the truck brought free cigarette samples. 'It looked like a Frosty truck,' Adamson said. 'I just remember people clamoring and cigarettes being handed out.'"

One of those children running to the cigarette truck was Marie Evans, who was given free cigarettes as a 9-year-old in Boston's Orchard Park. Marie died of lung cancer at age 54. Her son, Willie Evans, sued the makers of Newport cigarettes, Lorillard Tobacco Company, and in 2010 a Massachusetts court awarded the Evans family more than $180 million in damages. The jury ruled the tobacco company gave out free cigarettes in Black neighborhoods to entice Black children to become smokers. The company denied the claims.

Where you live is an indicator of your education and employment. How much you earn and when you quit school are as strongly associated with dangerous blood sugar levels in diabetics as clinical risk factors. If you live in an area packed with fast food restaurants and corner shops that sell sugary snacks, not vegetables, you are more likely to be diagnosed with type 2 diabetes than someone who lives in an area with grocers and farmers' markets. Where you live matters more than your genes.

More than 23 million Americans live in food deserts, places where a supermarket or large grocery store is more than a mile away, according to the US Department of Agriculture. Take a map, outline the areas that are food deserts, and you will find they overlap with areas that are health care deserts, places where health care is hard to get to or nonexistent. A shortage of primary care doctors is especially apparent, which is worrying, since these doctors focus on preventive care and routine monitoring such as blood pressure and blood sugar.

Zip codes where mostly Black and Hispanic people live are more likely to have a shortage of primary care doctors, according to a study by researchers at Johns Hopkins Bloomberg School of Public Health. They defined a shortage as either no primary care doctor at all or one primary care doctor for more than 3,500 people.

A quarter of African Americans and 24.3 percent of Hispanic people lived in zip codes with either no primary care doctors or very few. That was compared to 13.2 percent of whites and 9.6 percent of Asians.

In a map of the United States zigzagged with bright orange lines and short blue and purple dashes, data scientist Sohan Murthy creates a visual representation of the country's health care deserts. Using information from an online database of nearly a million doctors, Murthy looked at Americans' accessibility to obstetricians and gynecologists, radiation oncologists, and emergency medicine doctors. His map shows that many health care deserts overlap with actual deserts—across the Sonoran Desert of Arizona, the Mojave Desert of Nevada, across large swathes of eastern and southern Texas, and as far north as Washington and North Dakota.

There are 48,000 obstetricians and gynecologists practicing in 22,000 locations across the United States, Murthy tells us. That's almost the same number of emergency medicine doctors—49,000 working in 16,000 locations. But in many parts of the country, women have to travel farther to see a women's health doctor than to see an emergency medicine doctor, Murthy says.

His map shows the problem is worse for women living in the southeastern United States, a region that overlaps with the 200 mostly Black counties in the South known as the Black Belt.

Inequalities overlapped with inequalities. Poor communities with limited access to fresh foods and doctors. We're now shifting the blame away from individuals to look at maps that explain why some people live a decade less than others and suffer multiple chronic conditions (though there shouldn't have been any finger pointing in the first place, not unless those fingers were being pointed at politicians who enact policies that perpetuate the inequalities).

Digital maps, technology such as geographic information systems that manage spatial data, as well as datasets on income and occupation can be combined to create a person's ZNA. Much as we sequence genes to look for genetic mutations and risk factors for inherited disorders in DNA, we can use these data to sequence people's likelihood of suffering diabetes, depression, and lead poisoning, and to predict their life expectancy from the moment they are born—all based on their zip code.

46

Does debunking a myth help it spread?

ost-truth was the Oxford dictionary's word of the year in 2016. It defined *post-truth* as "relating to or denoting circumstances in which objective facts are less influential in shaping public opinion than appeals to emotion and personal belief." The word has been around for decades, but there was a spike in the use of *post-truth* in 2016 especially during the US presidential election and after Britain's vote to leave the European Union. *Post-truth politics* and *we're living in a post-truth world* have become popular phrases.

So what use is the truth anyway?

In 2014, Dr. Gary Freed, a pediatrician at the University of Michigan in Ann Arbor took more than 1,700 parents and split them into four groups. One group was shown photos of a toddler whose skin was covered in the red rash of measles, another child, a young boy whose cheeks and jaw were swollen from infection with mumps virus, and a baby, its face dotted with the red dots of a rubella rash, a hospital wrist band around its tiny arm and an IV line poking out of its frail body.

A second group of parents was given information debunking the claim that vaccines cause autism. A third group was told the potential side effects of the measles, mumps, and rubella vaccine. And the fourth group was given the story of a mother whose young son got so sick with measles that he had to spend time in the hospital.

Freed and his team had already asked the parents a series of questions about whether they had vaccinated their children, if they ever delayed or refused vaccines, and what they thought of the measles, mumps, and rubella (MMR) vaccine. After giving the groups their various pieces of information, Freed's team asked the parents again what they thought of the MMR vaccine and if they would vaccinate their children in the future.

The results might shock you.

Parents who were shown photos of sick children suffering with vaccine-preventable diseases doubled down on their belief that vaccines cause autism. Parents told the story of another parent's nightmare about a young boy being hospitalized with measles doubled down on their beliefs that vaccines cause severe side effects. Those given information debunking the claim that vaccines cause autism said they were less likely to vaccinate their children in the future. And information on the potential side effects of the MMR vaccine did not have a significant effect in swaying parents to like or dislike vaccines more than they did at the beginning of the experiment.

If that makes you want to throw your hands in the air and give up, wait for this: the next year, researchers at the University of Illinois at Urbana-Champaign used the very same photos of sick children in their study of attitudes toward vaccines.

They saw very different results.

They took 315 people (parents and nonparents), divided them into three groups, and used the exact same photos and text that Freed had used in his study a year earlier. One group was shown the same photos of children sick with MMR, the same mother's story of her son who became very sick with measles, and some warnings about MMR. Another group was given information proving that vaccines do not cause autism, and a third group was given scientific literature that had nothing to do with vaccines.

This time around, parents shown photos of children suffering with vaccine-preventable diseases looked at vaccines in a more favorable light after seeing the photos of sick children. The group given information that vaccines do not cause autism showed no difference in their attitudes toward vaccines.

These results are more optimistic for those who want to remain hopeful that facts can lead people to change their minds, but, before you get too excited, I should tell you this: In the second experiment, parents who were swayed to look at vaccines in a more favorable light after being given one of the interventions, well, they were already on the fence about vaccines. They didn't hold extremely negative views about vaccines to begin with.

For the rest, those who doubled down on their antivaccine views even after looking at photos of babies in incubators, a phenomenon known as the backfire effect might be at play.

The backfire effect says people become even more entrenched in their beliefs after being presented with factual information that goes against their personal beliefs. It says that presenting people with facts runs the risk of pushing them to create counterarguments against the facts and makes them burrow deeper into their own incorrect beliefs.

The backfire effect has been documented in all sorts of situations, including politics. In 2010 two political scientists, Jason Reifler and Brendan Nyhan, were studying political misperceptions and the likelihood that correcting a fake claim might change a person's mind. But when they showed people mock news articles saying weapons of mass destruction had been found in Iraq plus a correction saying this was an error and that no WMDs were discovered, they found that corrections didn't reduce misperceptions. In fact, corrections "actually *increase* misperceptions," they said. People became more convinced that WMDs had been found even though the correction said otherwise.

If debunking a claim makes some people double down on personal beliefs, such as the belief that vaccines cause autism, should we avoid repeating those claims in efforts to disprove them? It seems as if offering evidence against a conspiracy theory makes some people believe the conspiracy really is true. Or, as Reifler and Nyhan said, "Corrections frequently fail to reduce misperceptions."

It's not a newly documented phenomenon. It was studied in the 1950s by psychologists Leon Festinger, Stanley Schacter, and Henry Riecken, who described it this way in their book, *When Prophecy Fails:* "A man with a conviction is a hard man to change. Tell him you disagree and he turns away. Show him facts or figures and he questions your sources. Appeal to logic and he fails to see your point."

They go on to describe the doubling down of beliefs, the same phenomenon studied more recently by Reifler and Nyhan. "Suppose that he is presented with evidence, unequivocal and undeniable evidence, that his belief is wrong: what will happen? The individual will frequently emerge, not only unshaken, but even more convinced of the truth of his beliefs than ever before."

Debating a false claim might give it legitimacy and oxygen. Feels like a lose-lose situation. Should you even be reading this book? Should I have written it?

But in a paper titled "The Elusive Backfire Effect," two political scientists contradicted their colleagues. Thomas Wood and Ethan Porter enrolled more than 10,000 people and conducted five experiments on fifty-two polarizing issues—the kinds of topics where you might expect to see a backfire effect.

The result: "Across all experiments, we found no corrections capable of triggering backfire." Wood and Porter urged us not to worry too much. "Evidence of factual backfire is far more tenuous than prior research suggests. By and large, citizens heed factual information, even when such information challenges their ideological commitments."

Phew.

But there might be something else to worry about: the pushback effect. This is the idea that while we may not make up counterarguments against the facts, we still push back against the facts and dig deep into our own beliefs. The pushback effect is a concept explored by Eileen Dombrowski, author of the book *The Theory of Knowledge*.

While we think of beliefs about vaccines and health as deeply personal beliefs linked to very personal choices—should I vaccinate *my* kid? Should I feed *my* baby genetically modified foods?—false beliefs are very much a social and cultural phenomenon. They are often false beliefs that we share with friends, family, and neighbors. Shared beliefs are the glue of community; they confirm our place, our membership, and belonging. And because belonging is deeply important to humans, beliefs can feel like life or death. Not to mention the impact of not vaccinating your child spreads far wider than your family and affects your entire community.

Sometimes we believe a thing because it is the only explanation, or the simplest explanation, on offer. Think back to the chapter about the food additive monosodium glutamate and beliefs that it caused an illness called Chinese Restaurant Syndrome. It didn't. But availability heuristic, the idea that we come to conclusions using information that's easiest to find and we don't consider other explanations, could have been at play in that situation.

Those false beliefs about monosodium glutamate might have been legitimized by Chinese restaurant owners, who, in the fight to keep their businesses afloat, began writing "No MSG used here" in their menus. As if that was a good thing. It's a lot like when the Food and Drug Administration removed the preservative thimerosal from vaccines in 2001 on the recommendation of organizations such as the American Academy of Pediatrics. It was hoped that its removal would convince more people to get vaccinated. It's unlikely thimerosal removal increased vaccination rates. But for many its removal created an impression of risk. The FDA's actions were confirmation that the preservative must have been unsafe in the first place. Why else would a public health agency remove something from vaccines?

Would it have been easier to ignore concerns about monosodium glutamate and thimerosal? While some argue we should simply disregard fake news, that doesn't make the fake news go away. And, there is evidence that debunking a myth really can change people's minds. But how we do this is up for debate.

For some, facts are enough. To which I say, whose facts are they anyway? Let's list some of the facts that we don't talk about: 200 children were paralyzed in a 1955 polio vaccination program, tens of thousands of women were forcibly sterilized in American hospitals in the twentieth century, doctors working for the US government infected Guatemalans with gonorrhea. We don't talk much about the bloody history of public health or the creation of modern medicine. (That speculum your gynecologist uses was invented by a man who tested his inventions on enslaved women. He also performed experimental vaginal surgeries on enslaved women who were wide awake and not given anesthesia.)

By airing our dirty laundry, we get to the truth of modern-day public health travesties: why a tuberculosis outbreak might rage through twenty-first century Alabama, why the Nation of Islam is able to convince African American parents that vaccines are poison, why so few participants in clinical trials are people of color.

I began writing about this history and its impact on modern medicine in 2016 in a newspaper column called "Debunked." Soon after the column was launched in the *Dallas Morning News,* a reader wrote to say my headlines should not be phrased as questions because that raised the possibility of debate where there might not be one. I agreed with that reasoning and was swayed to change the format. "No, Trauma Is Not Inherited" and "Study Does Not Prove Diet Soda Causes Alzheimer's or Stroke" stood in place of headlines that would have been written as questions.

But I have changed my mind. While writing this book I sifted through the evidence about how we shape and shift personal beliefs, how we weigh new facts against long-held personal beliefs, and how we come to conclusions. Reading studies by philosophers, psychologists, epidemiologists, and political scientists, I decided that chapter titles framed as questions did not run the risk of stoking conspiracy theories.

I could be wrong. But like the photos of sick children that swayed some parents to vaccinate their own kids and caused others to double down on their antivaccine beliefs, the evidence is mixed.

We do know that some people are more susceptible to information disorder. Communities most vulnerable to infectious diseases are the same communities left vulnerable to fake news about health and science. On maps, health deserts—areas with few or no clinics—overlap with news deserts—places where local newspapers and radio stations have shuttered and communities are left with little access to reliable, life-saving information.

Nowadays I combine my training in medicine and journalism to track the spread of contagious misinformation about health as well as the spread of diseases. The two go hand in hand. Misinformation (fake news spread without the intention of causing harm), disinformation (fake news spread deliberately to hurt people), and malinformation (genuine information such as leaked emails and private documents that are weaponized to hurt people), spread alongside disease epidemics. Collectively they are known as information disorder, a term coined by Claire Wardle, director of the nonprofit news organization, First Draft News.

Information disorder fuels the spread of infections such as Ebola, measles, and flu. The spread of microbes and rumors about microbes bear uncanny similarities. In fact, when we map the spread of a rumor, we use the same models invented in the 1960s and 1970s to track the spread of infections. The similarities between contagious rumors and contagious microbes don't end there.

One of the first steps in an outbreak investigation involves going door to door in a neighborhood to find out who is sick, who knows someone who is sick, and who has been in contact with whom. Disease detectives use that information to make a spider's web network of all the cases and all the contacts. Sometimes you identify a person responsible for passing on the infection to many more people than the average infected person; we call these people superspreaders. Maybe because of their lifestyle or their genes, they are more contagious than most. The 20/80 rule says that in some outbreaks, 80 percent of cases are transmitted by 20 percent of people.

The same can be said of rumor networks. There are rumor superspreaders who, because of their social media status or standing in a community, are able to transmit a rumor to many more people than the average person. There are also people known as stiflers. When the infection (or rumor!) gets to them, it stops and doesn't spread onward.

If there are so many similarities in the spread of information disorder and infections, why not treat them in the same way? During an epidemic of disease, we use vaccines to protect people from becoming part of the outbreak. We might be able to do the same with fake news—we can try to inoculate against the spread of mistruths in just the way we inoculate against the spread of disease.

A theory from the world of social psychology uses a biological analogy to think about protection from rumors. Vaccines, such as the flu vaccine, inoculate us with a weakened version of the flu virus so that our immune system can learn to recognize the infection and be ready to mount a response. In that same way, inoculation theory says you can protect against the spread of fake news by preemptively exposing people to weakened rumors so that they build up mental immunity against attempts to deceive them. Preempting the fake news and neutralizing it is called prebunking. Based on the idea that it's easier to fool someone than it is to convince someone they have been fooled, prebunking prepares people for fake news by making them aware of the threat and offering a countermessage. It says, "Look out! Fake news on climate change or vaccine science or chemtrails is on its way! And here's why the messaging you are about to see is wrong."

"Inoculation messages have been found to be more effective at conveying resistance to misinformation than supportive messages (i.e., messages that promote accurate information without mentioning the misinformation)," wrote researchers at the Center for Climate Change Communication in Virginia in 2017.

In their study with collaborators in the United Kingdom and Australia, they tested inoculation theory to see if it neutralized misinformation about climate change. They inoculated one group with either a warning about misinformation or an explanation of why the news they would read was inaccurate. Another group was given both the warning and the explanation, and the control group was exposed to misinformation with no warning and no explanation.

Prebunking worked. Preemptively explaining misleading news neutralized its negative impact. The best protection was an explanation of exactly how the misinformation would be formatted and how it would try to dupe the reader.

This might work for fake news on climate change and vaccines, but what about the mis-, dis-, and malinformation that we don't see coming? A rumor about a made-up disease or rehashing of an old debate. Who thought that in 2018 there would be a vigorous debate about the earth being flat?! How can you prebunk against that?

But Melisa Basol, a social psychologist at the University of Cambridge, says: "You'd be surprised how many absurd arguments scholars have inoculated against so far, ranging from cultural truisms such as the benefits of brushing teeth, to animal testing, climate denialism, and stage fright, to name a few." Basol warns that misinformation "travels faster and farther than any other kind of information, making fact-checking an ambitious and somewhat naïve attempt to combat the societal challenges posed by misinformation."

Two years after *post-truth* was declared the Oxford dictionary's word of the year, Dictionary.com announced its word of the year: *misinformation*. "Our Word of the Year choice serves as a symbol of each year's most meaningful events and lookup trends," it said.

Facts are the universal antidote to misinformation, according to many science and health officials. I disagree. We must go beyond facts. If the conspiracy theories I grew up with were fascinating *because* they were fantastical, memorable *because* they were absurd, then facts—straight-up, clinical, sterile, facts—are not cutting it.

Neuroscience can help guide us through this dilemma. In his studies of the impact of stories on the brain, neuroscientist Paul Zak discovered that stories full of suspense, heartache, intrigue, and inspiration, cause the release of the neurotransmitter and hormone oxytocin. Stories have the power to expand our minds, shift our beliefs, and even change our behaviors.

The stories really do have to be compelling though. A video of a father embracing his two-year-old son who has terminal cancer and not much time left to live, caused oxytocin release in people watching the short film. After they had watched the emotional film, they were more likely to offer money to a stranger. The same effect was not seen when participants watched a video of the same father and son at the zoo. Cancer was not mentioned in that clip.

There's much more to be discovered about the effect of stories on our brains. But those primitive, sit around the fireplace, make me laugh/make me cry tales might hold the key to countering untruths about health and science. Facts are not enough. Facts don't seem to change minds; stories possess that power. At least that is the story I keep telling myself, the personal belief I am doubling down on, or maybe it is more hope than belief. A hope I need to believe because I don't want to live in a post-truth, misinformed world.

DR. YASMIN'S BULLSHIT DETECTION KIT
Cut out and keep!

In a world brimming with hoaxes and rapidly changing information, here's your protection against false news. Inspired by Carl Sagan's book chapter "The Fine Art of Baloney Detection," Dr. Yasmin's Bullshit Detection Kit is a twenty-first-century shield against scientific lies. Like Carl Sagan, I want to help you find a balance between healthy skepticism and an open mind. Here's what to ask when weighing the credibility of news headlines, scientific papers, tweets, and watercooler chitchat.

---

1. Who is making the claim? Have they been reliable in the past? Do their peers trust them—even the ones who might disagree with them?

---

2. If an image is part of the claim, use a reverse search engine to check the provenance of the image. Has it been doctored in any way? Do earlier versions of the image or video look different from what's being shared? Be wary of viral videos. Use tools like Amnesty International's DataViewer, which tells you when the video was uploaded. Other tools can help you trace the provenance of photos or videos. The person who uploaded the photo or video might not be the same person who shot the photo or video. Search for the original source.

---

3. Follow the money: Look at the person making the claim and ask, who pays them? Don't just look at salaries, look at grants, outside funding, and their investments to search for potential financial motivations. (Andrew Wakefield, the discredited British doctor who made up science about the MMR vaccine, had undisclosed business dealings set to potentially earn him millions of pounds if he was able to discredit the MMR vaccine and guide people toward his "replacement vaccine" and autism businesses. We learned of Wakefield's financial dealings thanks to investigative journalist Brian Deer.)

4. Who benefits, who is hurt? Does the information being shared harm anyone's credibility, livelihood, or health? Who might be out to get that person or community? If someone or some organization looks to benefit, ask questions about their role in propagating the information. Is a study about the health benefits of vitamin D sponsored by a vitamin D manufacturer or lobbying group? Look for a debate on the claim by people with various perspectives.

5. Common sense: Weird things happen and weirdness lends itself to virality, but is what you're seeing or hearing credible? Does it fit into the way the world works?

6. Don't get overly attached to one hypothesis. Keep an open mind. Consider alternative theories.

7. Occam's razor: A philosophical principle that reminds us to keep things simple. If there are two or three explanations for something, consider the explanation that requires *fewest* assumptions.

8. Testing the claim: Can the findings be duplicated? Has anyone disproved the claim?

9. Are personal beliefs driving the claim?

10. Has the claim been verified by people or organizations who are not affiliated with the source?

11. If there are multiple links in the chain of an argument then each link must be held up to scrutiny.

---

12. Question authority: Governments have made mistakes and intentionally and unintentionally harmed people. Look for independent experts to back up the claims of authorities.

ACKNOWLEDGMENTS

Thank you to my editors at the *Dallas Morning News,* who stoked my enthusiasm for debunking medical myths and pseudoscience and encouraged me to begin a newspaper column called "Debunked." Many of the chapters in this book began as columns, which were lovingly edited by Mede Nix. Thank you, Mede, for entertaining my ideas about cat poop and encouraging me to write stories about placenta parties and other weird behaviors. (But it was always clear that the cat poop story was your favorite!) Thank you to readers of the *Dallas Morning News* and to my Twitter followers, who continue to send me questions for debunking. Much love to Tristan Brown for discussions about Carl Sagan and the idea for a modern take on the baloney detection kit. Science journalist extraordinaire, Lauren Silverman, contributed to reporting on thalidomide and aspirin's Nazi connection when we worked together on a podcast called *Drugged.* Thanks to Melisa Basol for careful reading of portions of the manuscript and expert guidance on inoculation theory. Finally, thank you to the peer reviewers who provided thoughtful comments on the book.

ABOUT THE AUTHOR

Seema Yasmin is a medical doctor, poet, professor, and professional debunker. She is director of the Stanford Center for Health Communication and a clinical assistant professor in the Stanford University School of Medicine. Yasmin teaches science journalism and global health storytelling and studies the spread of microbes and misinfodemics. Born in Nuneaton, Warwickshire, and raised in Hackney, London, she lives in California with her pit bull, Lily.

Submit suspected health hoaxes and general inquiries via the contact form at www.seemayasmin.com.

ALSO BY THE AUTHOR:

The Impatient Dr. Lange: One Man's Fight to End the Global HIV Epidemic

Muslim Women Are Everything: Stereotype-Shattering Stories of Courage, Inspiration, and Adventure

If God Is a Virus: The Ebola Poems

INDEX

abortion: availability of, 72–73

absolute risk. *See* relative risk vs. absolute risk

accidental poisoning, 9–10

acesulfame-K, 57

acetylsalicylic acid, 84. *See also* aspirin

activated charcoal: as detox, 10; as remedy for accidental poisoning, 10

acute flaccid myelitis (AFM), 30–32, 37–38; and EV-D68, 31–32, 33, 36–38; possible causes of, 31–32, 35; prevalence of, 31, 32; prevention of, 38; prognosis for, 31

Adamson, Leslie, 234

aegeline: as unsafe ingredient, 107–8

African Americans: as blood donors, 111–12. *See also* race; racism

AIDS epidemic. *See* HIV/AIDS epidemic

airline industry, 214. *See also* contrails/chemtrails

alcohol: as harmful to a fetus, 190; as risk factor for breast cancer, 64

Alzheimer's disease: artificial sweeteners as risk factor for, 55–58; symptoms of, 55

Ambien, 223

Amin, Iftekhar, 184

amygdala: and implicit bias, 224

antibiotics: fears over, 4

antidepressants: as treatment for multiple health issues, 89

antivaccine movement, 238–39; dangers of, 17–24

Arctic apples, 46

artificial sweeteners: as risk factor for stroke and dementia, 55–58

asbestos: as cause of mesothelioma, 168; and talcum powder, 167–69

aspartame, 57; risks associated with, 56

aspartic acid, 56

aspirin: as cancer preventative, 78–81; and cardiovascular disease, 81; origins of, 83–84; popularity of, 82; side effects of, 82. *See also* Bayer

astute clinician method, 189–90

athletic performance: effect of cannabis on, 121–24

atypical hyperplasia, 64

Augustine, Norman, 153

Autism Education Summit, 26

autism spectrum disorder (ASD): fake treatments for, 25–29; among Somali American children, 19; prevalence of, 25, 27; vaccines believed to be a cause of, 17–18, 19, 21

Autistic Rights Together, 28

availability heuristic, 52–53, 241

backfire effect, 239–40

Badu, Erykah, 229

Baldor, Daniel, 213

Barr, Roseanne, 223

Basol, Melisa, 244

Bassuk, Shari S., 95

Bayer (firm), historical ties to Nazi Germany, 83–86

Beck (musician), 229

beta blockers, 223. *See also* propanolol

Bhutanese refugees: suicide among, 198–99

birth control pills: and risk of depression, 87–91

birth defects: resulting from thalidomide, 125–33; and Zika virus, 187, 189–92

bisexual men. *See* gay and bisexual men

Black babies: mortality rate for, 71

Black people: impact of stress on their health, 69–70

Black women: maternal mortality rate, 67, 69

Blau, Abram, 158

bleach, industrial: as fake treatment for autism, 26, 28, 29

blood donation: from gay and bisexual men, 110–14; from Haitian Americans, 113; and infectious diseases, 113; racial profiling in, 111–12

blood shortages, 111

Borkin, Joseph, 85